Praise for Aimee Raupp

Aimee Raupp is one of the most kind, generous, and talented healers. Her ability to hold her patients with love and compassion is her greatest strength. Aimee has transformed the way I think about my body and my healing path. Not only is she an incredible acupuncturist, but she's an undercover therapist too! The moment you walk into Aimee's office, you feel like you're wrapped in a warm blanket of love.

— **Gabrielle Bernstein**, NY Times Best-selling author, international speaker & Spirit Junkie

Aimee is the perfect mix between fertility expert meets acupuncturist meets therapist. I am so grateful to have her in my life for her guidance and knowledge. She has really helped me through my fertility journey in a way I didn't know I needed.

— **Hannah Bronfman**, Author, health & wellness enthusiast, founder of hbfit.com

Aimee Raupp is a leading expert in women's health and fertility, leveraging her deep understanding of Eastern and Western medicine and decades of clinical experience to improve outcomes in even the most complex cases. I consider her to be an invaluable partner and regularly recommend patients incorporate her treatments and philosophies into their care plans.

— **Frank Lipman**, M.D. NY Times Best-selling author & Head of Functional Medicine at The Well

Aimee is a beacon of hope for all looking to improve their health and awaken their best life.

— **Deepak Chopra**, M.D., Best-selling author, public speaker & alternative medicine advocate

I would only send my patients struggling with fertility to see Aimee Raupp and her team for help with their diet AND LIFESTYLE. Together with PRP Ovarian Rejuvenation, the Egg Quality Diet in this book can do magic to those struggling with poor egg quality.

— **Zaher Merhi**, M.D., HCLD, Medical Director, RFC

THE EGG QUALITY DIET:

A clinically proven 100-day fertility diet to balance hormones, reduce inflammation, improve egg quality & optimize your ability to get & stay pregnant

Aimee E. Raupp, M.S., L. Ac.

Best-selling author of Yes, You Can Get Pregnant, natural fertility expert, acupuncturist & herbalist

To you and your dream baby.
To the hope in your heart.
To your tenacity.
May all your dreams come true.

Testimonials for *The Egg Quality Diet*

At the moment, I am 43 and almost 17 weeks pregnant and have been cautiously optimistic because we lost our last pregnancy due to chromosomal abnormality. After losing that pregnancy, we went on the roller coaster ride of fertility treatments, all unsuccessful. During that time, I happened to come across Aimee's books as recommended by another fertility group that I participate in. I could not put them down. Through them, I have learned so much about diet, emotions, and myself. I wholeheartedly implemented all her recommendations. We were prepping for our last embryo transfer, scheduled for, and I felt so good and healthy on Aimee's program that my husband and I decided to try naturally. We got pregnant NATURALLY on our second month trying! Because I had been following Aimee's program for 6 months, we never needed the IVF transfer! I still cannot BELIEVE that I got pregnant naturally after several failed IVFs! I feel so blessed to have this opportunity and am very thankful for Aimee, and her wisdom, love, and support, which I know has gotten me on this path, one that I never thought I would experience, let alone naturally!

—M.F., 43

So my egg retrieval is all over, and we ended up with 14 embryos making it to blast! I really do think The Egg Quality Diet helped me! As this is my 3rd IVF retrieval in 2 years, and I'm now 39 and have never had such amazing results. We have 5 normal embryos from this batch!

—J.S., 39

I am currently 20 weeks pregnant with a healthy baby, and I would not have been able to get and stay pregnant if it weren't for what I learned from Aimee Raupp and her teachings, especially the nutrition piece. Aimee's expertise and encouragement guided me through overhauling my entire lifestyle, and as a result, I got pregnant, two months before my 44th birthday, after five losses, and without IVF.

—K.P., 44

We had TWO euploids for this round!!! My Dr. was worried we wouldn't get any normal embryos. For a total of 3 (including the one from the last round). I am so happy. I can't believe we have these three beautiful embryos. I am so used to being in this space of IVF retrievals and getting no embryos, let alone PGS tested NORMALS! And, now entering a new phase of transferring, which is scary! I know I CAN get pregnant, and now we have these healthy embryos to transfer. I know this diet had everything to do with it! Thank you, thank you!

—B. L., 36

After several failed IVF cycles, resulting in ZERO genetically normal embryos, I dived wholeheartedly into Aimee's diet, and I am proud to say that we just had another IVF cycle and got our FIRST healthy embryo! I am so grateful to Aimee for all her guidance.

—T.C., 42

I found Aimee two years into our TTC journey when I had really lost all hope in my ability to get pregnant and have a healthy pregnancy (3 miscarriages, 4 failed IVF's, so much heartache). I had nearly given up entirely as I felt like I was doing EVERYTHING, and nothing was working. That is when my friend urged me to reach out and work with Aimee. I wasn't happy about it, but I said, fine, what do I have to lose. What I really should have said was what do I have to gain. The answer: Everything. Aimee brought me back to life. From our first meeting, she drilled down into my lifestyle and made immediate changes. Aimee gave me hope. Something I hadn't felt in a really long time. I responded to her by being 100% committed to her plan and did everything she suggested, from using Ghee to switching to healthy beauty products to making organic bone broth. I started eating FAT, and I actually started to lose weight. I meditated and exercised. He then suggested and focused on my health and well-being. The shift happened about a month after seeing Aimee. I started to feel lighter, happier, more confident in myself. I was a new, improved person, and I loved the new me. As I type this, I'm now 25 weeks pregnant, and I'm grateful every day for Aimee's rock-solid support, guidance, and encouragement. Aimee believed in me, and that made me believe in myself.

—R.M., 44

Deciding to finally reach out and work with Aimee was one of the smartest decisions I made on my fertility journey - which eventually led to my healthy baby boy. She redirected all of the pent-up guilt I had acquired on the fertility journey about what I should/shouldn't eat - and instead - helped me to focus on what really mattered. Which was making conscious choices both physically and mentally that would make me feel good every day. Not just so that I could get pregnant. Deciding to trust and surrender to her guidance made me feel like I had someone on my side. She doesn't make you feel like a patient.

She sees you as a friend and a person who has been through a lot. And I felt seen and heard, which is so needed when TTC. She is so easy to work with and smart as hell. I highly recommend hiring her to walk with you and relieve you from feeling like you have to do this all on your own!

—S. B., 31

I've been following Aimee's recommendations and have been on the fertility-boosting diet for a few months. I noticed physical improvements soon after I made dietary changes and started taking the recommended supplements. Physically, I've never felt better. Thank you, Aimee! I have faith in my mind, body, and spirit once again!!!

—C.G., 39

From 2013 until early 2018, I was a shadow of myself. That's five years. Five years of heartbreak, grief, and straight-up medical neglect. I gave birth to my daughter in 2012 and, in an effort for a second baby, had four consecutive and "unexplained" miscarriages. I began working with a Reproductive Immunologist, Dr. Braverman, and I was diagnosed with endometriosis and PCOS. As a result of an inflammation level over the 90th percentile, he said I needed to give up gluten and then suggested I seek additional advice from Aimee Raupp, a trusted friend and Women's Wellness Expert. When I took Aimee's symptoms questionnaire, I was staggered to see that I had FORTY-TWO symptoms of autoimmunity and inflammation. I had forty-two symptoms and about as many Doctors' reports saying I was healthy. In my heart, I knew that I was finally finding the answers I'd needed for years. I began following her on Facebook and tuning in for her weekly live videos, which normally discussed fertility, wellness, mindset, and overall lifestyle. I signed up for a free phone consult with Aimee and felt so connected to her. She recommended that I dive into her diet plan and assured me that I was not broken and I could heal. And so, that's exactly what I did. After a few tough weeks on the diet, I saw the shift. I felt incredible. I felt lighter, more energetic, clear-minded, and grounded. My grief, anxiety, and depression began to subside. I began to feel alive again for the first time in years. To say that Aimee has changed my life is an understatement of vast proportion. I cannot recommend her program enough and pray that all women on this lonely journey find the peace I have through Aimee's work. And, now I have a healthy baby girl in my arms to show for it.

—L. F., 34

Just before I discovered Aimee, I had fibroid surgery, and as my body was healing, my menstrual cycles were still irregular. I've always been proactive in taking care of my health, but I was really at a loss as to how to get my menstrual cycles back to normal and wondered if I even could. Then I discovered Aimee's and her teachings, and they changed my life! I began immediately implementing Aimee's recommendations, and my body began to feel like it was coming into balance again. Joint pain, circles under my eyes, hair loss, irregular cycles, all these issues began to disappear. And, shortly after implementing Aimee's dietary recommendations, my cycles became regular!

—D. C., 37

I found Aimee through her book, Yes You Can Get Pregnant after a failed IVF cycle, and I was so lost. My cycles were out of whack, I felt alone in my fertility struggles, my anxiety was *at an all-time high (though I always had issues with this), I was on medication for low thyroid levels, and I was a teacher, I wasn't putting any time into taking care of myself. After finding Aimee, everything changed because I was prioritizing myself first. Aimee's plan pushed me to make big changes to my diet and supplements, as well as journal, meditate, and spend more time in nature. The biggest changes for me were my thyroid normalized on its own without medication after completing Aimee's Egg Quality diet. And, after several IVF cycles resulting in zero normal embryos, I finally went on to make some healthy embryos (thanks to Aimee's diet plan), and I am FINALLY pregnant with a healthy, thriving baby.*

—A. M., 36

I am 31 years old, and at 29 I found out my FSH was in the 50's. I was told I was in premature menopause. I was devastated. But I just knew there was something I could do to turn this around. This couldn't be my fate. That's when I found Aimee. I started following Aimee's diet plan right away (and doing the emotional work too). Within 9 months on her plan, my FSH now ranges between a 9 and a 12. I am not yet pregnant, but I know I will be soon, and Aimee's diet made all the difference. I am forever grateful.

—M.B., 31

I found Aimee through Dr. Braverman as I'd asked him specifically about nutrition, knowing that it was one of the things in my fertility journal that made me most anxious. I had 3 early miscarriages of genetically normal embryos prior to starting with Braverman and constantly feared how what I was eating or not eating affected eggs, embryos, and pregnancies. Google, friends and family, and fertility support groups offered conflicting advice and what worked for one person was the opposite of what worked for another. Something told me to do what Aimee said as she had so much success with women like me. I dove into all of Aimee's advice, and within 18 months of following her advice I was holding in my arms my very own beautiful baby girl.

— S. A., 42

Table of Contents:

About The Author

Aimee Raupp, MS, LAc, is a renowned women's health & fertility expert, celebrity acupuncturist & coach, and the best-selling author of the books *Chill Out & Get Healthy*, *Yes, You Can Get Pregnant*, and *Body Belief*. Aimee works virtually with clients worldwide, as well she is a licensed acupuncturist and herbalist in private practice in New York and Connecticut. Aimee holds a Master of Science degree in Traditional Oriental Medicine from the Pacific College of Oriental Medicine and a Bachelor's degree in biology from Rutgers University. Aimee's work in helping women transform their health and fertility has been supported by multiple Reproductive Endocrinologists and Medical Doctors. Aimee is also the founder of the Aimee Raupp Beauty line of hand-crafted, organic skincare products that are optimized for hormone harmony. She has appeared on *The View*, and has been featured in *Glamour*, *Allure*, *Well + Good*, *Mind Body Green*, *GOOP*, *Shape*, and many podcasts, including *Wellness Mama, Melissa Ambrosini, and Dr. Frank Lipman*. Aimee has received endorsements from Dr. Deepak Chopra, Dr. Frank Lipman, Arianna Huffington, Hannah Bronfman, and Gabrielle Bernstein for her work in helping thousands of women to improve their fertility, celebrate their beauty, and reconnect to the presence of their optimal health. In addition to working alongside several reproductive endocrinologists in the New York and Connecticut area, Aimee is also the Head of Chinese Medicine at The Well in NYC and is a frequent speaker at women's health & wellness conferences across the nation. She engages her large community worldwide through her social media presence, online programs, and her website, www.aimeeraupp.com.

Preface: How This Book Will Help You

~~~~~~~~~~~

"You have the power to change your health
& improve your fertility."
-Yes, You Can Get Pregnant

~~~~~~~~~~~

Have you tried everything to get pregnant, and nothing seems to work? Has your doctor told you the eggs in your ovaries are all bad? Or that donor egg is your only option for having a baby? Have you done multiple rounds of fertility treatments with no baby to show for it? Are you worried you're too old to have a baby? Have you spent half your paycheck on antioxidant vitamins and fertility smoothie ingredients and still have no idea how or why they can help you get pregnant? Do you feel overwhelmed by all the information out there on improving your fertility?

If so, you are in the right place.

I am Aimee Raupp. People call me a fertility detective because I am really, really good at figuring out the *why* behind a woman's fertility challenges and what she needs to do to fix them. I have been in the business of helping women get pregnant for 17 years as a practitioner of Traditional Chinese Medicine (TCM), acupuncturist, and herbalist. Before studying TCM, I was a biologist and neuroscience researcher. Over the years, I have written several books, helped thousands of babies come into this world, and continued my education in herbs, nutrition, neuroscience, and functional medicine. All of that means: I look at fertility through a different lens than most traditional western doctors do. Where many western doctors see fertility as being all about how many eggs you have left, your hormone levels, and your age, I know for certain, through all of my clinical experience, research, and continuing education, otherwise. Your fertility is an extension of your health. And when I say health, I mean it in a multifactorial way as health has physical, nutritional, mental-emotional, and environmental components, *all of which must be addressed for fertility to be recovered* (Yes, you can recover from your fertility challenges, and yes, you can improve your egg quality).

The Egg Quality Diet is the culmination of what I have found to be the most effective nutritional approach to optimizing fertility. This diet has been proven to work not in a randomized control trial (RCT) but in real life, on thousands of real women like you. Real women who have been told they have no good eggs left or they are too old or they are in menopause. This diet has been proven in women with high follicle-stimulating hormone (FSH), low anti-mullerian hormones (AMH), recurrent pregnancy loss (RPL), multiple failed in-vitro fertilizations (IVF), and intrauterine inseminations (IUI). This diet has been proven in women with endometriosis, polycystic ovarian syndrome (PCOS), fibroids, cysts, adenomyosis, asherman's syndrome, premature ovarian failure (POF), and hypothalamic amenorrhea. This diet has helped hundreds of women, even those in their mid to late forties, make healthy babies *using their own eggs*. This diet has helped women bring their FSH from above 50 down to 10. This diet has helped women double, even triple their AMH. Even more, this diet has been recommended by multiple reproductive endocrinologists (R.E.) to their clients mainly because, as one R.E. (the late Dr. Jeffrey Braverman) said to me, "I usually recommend a paleo or Mediterranean diet for my clients, but your diet is incredible. I've just never seen fertility improve so quickly. Whatever you are doing with your clients, keep doing it!"

What I offer you in this book is what I have clinically seen be effective for women trying to conceive. I can speak to the transformations I have repeatedly witnessed in my thousands of clients who follow this diet-- their hormones balance, their inflammatory markers improve, they make better quality embryos, and their fertility thrives. What once appeared to be a hopeless situation transforms into hope. I want that for you. I want you to get what you are worthy of-- that beautiful and healthy baby.

The one thing that is important to mention is that this book *only focuses on diet*. It does NOT focus on the other deeply important pillars of fertility rejuvenation which I have found to be: mental & emotional health, non-toxic lifestyle choices, supplements, movement, and sleep. Laced throughout this book (especially in Chapters 5 & 6), I will be giving you pointers on things like fertility supplements, tips for sperm health, genetic factors, non-toxic beauty products, and lifestyle adjustments you can make, but for a deep dive into all the ways you can support your fertility, I encourage you to check out my other books, namely: *Yes, You Can Get Pregnant* and *Body Belief*. As well, head over to AimeeRaupp.com/EQDiet and check out all the fertility resources I have put together for you there so you can get all the support you need on this challenging journey.

What Is *The Egg Quality Diet*

The Egg Quality Diet is a 100-day omnivorous eating plan based on my 17 years of clinical experience seeing what has worked time and time again for women. It is your ultimate roadmap to giving your body the nourishment it needs for your fertility to radically improve. In this book, I am giving you 100 days of menus, grocery shopping lists, recipes, hack sheets, and more. Literally, this book contains a step-by-step process to follow this diet so you can improve your egg quality and get pregnant with your dream baby. But before we dive into all of that, I want to talk to you about why this is the diet I have landed on and why it is different from many fertility diets out there, including the one I share in my best-selling book, *Yes, You Can Get Pregnant*.

When I wrote *Yes, You Can Get Pregnant* (one of the best-selling books on all things fertility), I included a meal plan that is much like the other fertility diets out there-- a mix of the Mediterranean and paleo diet with a strong focus on antioxidant-rich foods (like vegetables and fruit), good quality protein and fat. *That kind of diet definitely works for helping some women get pregnant.* So, don't fret if you've been following the *Yes, You Can Get Pregnant* diet, as that's still a great starting point, and it works for a lot of women. In fact, I still strongly recommend and consider *Yes, You Can Get Pregnant* to be one of the best and most comprehensive fertility books out there as it covers so much more than diet, so definitely give it a read if you haven't already. But, I have found clinically that the general paleo or Mediterranean fertility diet doesn't help ALL women. There are a few reasons why I believe this is happening:

- It can be too general, leaving room for error.
- Many of the women following these diets don't get the right macros (percentages of fat, protein, and carbs) for their fertility.
- Many of the women who have gone gluten-free eat too many processed, packaged, sugar-laden gluten-free foods and too many gluten-free grains.
- Many of the women following these diets are still suffering from inflammatory issues like PMS, heavy periods, clots with their periods, miscarriage, brain fog, headaches, fertility challenges, skin issues, gas, bloating, irregular bowel movements, low energy, and more.
- Many of these diets don't take into account gut dysbiosis and its impact on nutritional deficiencies impacting hormones and fertility.

- None of these fertility diets are elimination diets, which is absolutely key because every woman has a different body.
- Many of these diets don't stress that you can't out supplement an unbalanced, nutrient-poor diet. Even more, if you don't have optimal digestion (meaning- little to no gas or bloat and a healthy formed bowel movement one to two times per day) you're not absorbing nor getting benefit from those costly supplements if you can't absorb them.

The Egg Quality Diet solves all those problems. In this book, you will get 100 days of meal plans that are balanced for the ideal macros for fertility (more on this in the next chapter), powerfully anti-inflammatory and healing to your gut. Even more, you will be starting this diet off by eliminating any and all food groups that could be compromising your fertility. By starting *The Egg Quality Diet* with an elimination protocol, you will learn exactly the foods that your body doesn't react well to (think: foods that make you gassy, bloated, itchy, puffy, cause breakouts, headaches, brain fog, PMS, irregular periods and fatigue). You see, some women need to cut back on eating too many nuts, some can't have nightshade vegetables, some can't have beans, some need fewer grains, some need more, some can have gluten, some can't, some react fine to dairy and some don't. The beauty of this diet is you get to figure out what is right for you and your body. And, when you do that, you change your entire internal landscape on a cellular level; you heal your gut and begin digesting your food and absorbing all of your nutrition so that your body can do what it was meant to do-- grow a healthy baby.

In the pages that follow, I will dive a bit deeper into inflammation, autoimmunity, epigenetics, and gut health and why managing those conditions lay the ground for optimal fertility and egg quality. Before we get to that, I want to share my promise to you…

My Promise To You

I can't promise that making all the diet shifts I am recommending will be easy for you, but they will be worth it. I can't promise that at the end of the 100 days, you will be pregnant, but I can tell you that you will be closer than you are now, plus you'll have glowing skin, less bloat, and happier hormones. Yes, the upsides to this diet, besides better quality eggs, balanced hormones, and reduced inflammation, are less brain fog, better digestion, improved energy, healthier periods, juicier ovulations, little to no PMS, radiant skin, fewer aches and pains, fewer headaches and a more even-keeled you. My promise to you is that the way of eating mapped out in this book will give your body all the nutrition it needs to make a healthy, thriving baby, *and as a side effect, all the cells in your body will thrive too.*

I also want to promise you that on the resources page that goes with this book, AimeeRaupp.com/EQDiet, you will get so many additional tools to make this journey a success for you. It is with deep gratitude that I invite you to empower yourself with the knowledge herein and embrace this lifestyle as a means to improve your egg quality, your hormones, your uterine receptivity, and ultimately, your ability to conceive.

CHAPTER ONE

Can I Really Improve
The Quality Of My Eggs

There are many reasons to pick up a book on optimizing egg quality. Maybe you're trying to get pregnant now, maybe you've struggled with fertility challenges in the past and are looking to make some changes, maybe you're in the throes of fertility treatments and need more guidance on how to reduce inflammation or improve egg quality, maybe your FSH (follicle-stimulating hormone) is high, or your AMH (anti-mullerian hormones) is low, or your doctor told you that your eggs are all bad. Or perhaps it's that you have seen a friend or loved one go through fertility challenges and you are worried about the health of your eggs, maybe you have gone through one or more miscarriages and need a fresh perspective on how to approach your fertility, maybe you're in your 40's and want to do everything possible to optimize your health and fertility now, or maybe you want to know about how to preserve your fertility best and help your body now for a time in the future when you are ready to conceive. Whatever your reason for picking up this book, I know the diet in this book can help because it has been the cornerstone of the work I do, helping thousands of women all over the world get and stay pregnant with their own eggs.

I want to help you improve your health and optimize your fertility because I know that fertility struggles suck. Feeling disempowered and in doubt of your body and its state of health is emotionally draining. Not knowing where to turn to get reliable help can feel lonely. Feeling overwhelmed by worry over your ability to conceive when you want to is paralyzing. Being told by your doctor that your options are limited and your chances of conception are slim feels harrowing. It is for those reasons and more that I wrote this book. I want to inspire hope in your heart and remind you of the power you have over your health and fertility. From all of my experience working with women just like you: although we may not be able to change how many eggs you have left, I know we can improve the quality of those eggs.

With *The Egg Quality Diet*, my mission is to show you that choosing to consume anti-inflammatory, macronutrient balanced and nutrient-dense foods is hands down your best ally when making better quality eggs, balancing your hormones, and conceiving the healthy child you long for. My intention is that this book will be a roadmap to eating your way to a healthier, happier, more fertile you. My dream is that you will feel not only empowered after reading this book and adopting this way of eating but that you will confidently own your wellness as it is the basis of your fertility and your egg quality. It is truly my belief as a seasoned practitioner of nearly 20 years and a steadfast practice-r of what I preach that **you have the power to change your health and improve your fertility**. I wrote this book, *all of my books,* to remind you of that.

How do I know this dietary approach works? Because I have helped thousands of women conceive (just head to my website, AimeeRaupp.com, and read some of my Stories of Hope). And, by embracing this lifestyle myself, I conceived naturally and with ease at 40 years old, at 44 years old (sadly, I miscarried due to Turner's syndrome, which isn't age-related), and now at the age of 46, I still believe in the possibility of my getting pregnant again with a healthy child (and using my own eggs). I believe in it because I follow my own recommendations. P.S. I've had more than one

CAN I REALLY IMPROVE THE QUALITY OF MY EGGS?

fertility doctor tell me that I have the hormones and the ovaries of a woman five years my junior. I know this diet is the primary reason for that, and there's science presented in this book that will show you this way of living actually takes 3 + years off your physiological age (more on that in the pages that follow).

For all the other tools I use to maximize my fertility and the fertility of my clients, be certain to check out my other books: Yes, You Can Get Pregnant and Body Belief as well go to the resources page we have created to go in hand with this book: AimeeRaupp.com/EQDiet

But My Doctor Told Me
There Is No Hope With My Own Eggs

I hear this *all the time.*

"Aimee, my doctor said there is no hope. Can I really improve the quality of my eggs?"

You were probably told or read somewhere that you were born with all the eggs your ovaries will ever have. As far as we know, that is true (although there's some interesting research putting this theory into question[1]) however what we don't know much about scientifically, is the quality of those eggs. Even more, recent medical studies show that ovarian aging is more about mitochondrial function (aka cellular health) than it is about physiological age[2] (and all of my teachings will absolutely help you optimize cellular health and mitochondrial function). What we are taught is that as we age, the quality of the eggs in our ovaries declines. This is based on the notion that aging causes oxidation (a process similar to rusting, but it happens on the inside of our bodies at the cellular level) and oxidation negatively impacts cellular quality and mitochondrial health and when that happens, every single cell in your body, including the ones in your ovaries lose their vitality. What this translates to is: the older you are the less healthy the cells that make up the eggs in your ovaries are and hence the less likely they are to make a chromosomally normal baby. This theory is plausible however there are three big issues with this idea:

1. It doesn't account for epigenetics. Epigenetics is the study of how certain environmental factors (lifestyle, diet, mental-emotional state) impact how we age (or don't) on a cellular level.

2. It goes against other scientific notions that we can heal from disease, slow down the aging process and prevent or delay the onset of age related issues[3] (like the so-called inevitable decline of those eggs in your ovaries).

3. It doesn't address how co-existing health challenges (like autoimmunity and inflammation) are impacting fertility.

My approach to the aging egg discussion has always been based on the idea that if we can reverse heart disease or Type II diabetes or heal from cancer or any other disease, why on earth can't we recover our aging ovaries? It's really all the same thing. You see, we are made up of trillions of cells and science shows us that how we live our life-- the choices we make on a daily basis-- influences the overall state of inflammation and oxidation in our bodies. So by that train of thinking then what we do with our choices impact how those cells in our body--including the ones in your ovaries--decline or revitalize. And, this isn't just my clinical theory based on the thousands of transformations I have witnessed. There is very promising data supporting those anti-inflammatory and antioxidant agents (meaning supplements and dietary sources) positively impact how the eggs in your ovaries age[4]. As I stated on page 76 in my best-selling book, *Yes You Can Get Pregnant,* "scientific research presented at the Annual Clinical Meeting of the American College of Obstetricians and Gynecologists by Dr Jeffrey Russel, showed that a protein-rich diet is essential for good quality embryos and better egg quality. As well… several scientific articles have shown that antioxidants ward off oxidative stress (another term for premature aging) and improve both male and female fertility." Even more, research that came out after I wrote *Yes, You Can Get Pregnant* concluded that "in relation to the oxidative stress as a co-factor of defective oocyte maturation, an appropriate intake of proteins, antioxidants and methyl-donor supplements may decrease the bioavailability of toxic oxidants resulting in the protection of oocyte maturation."[5] Researchers in 2020 concluded in that, "The ovarian microenvironment and the stress that is induced by environmental pollutants and a poor diet, along with other factors, impact oocyte quality and function and contribute to accelerated oocyte aging and diseases of infertility"[6]. In other words, the scientific literature is showing that a diet high in antioxidants, protein and nutrient density improves egg quality and staves off ovarian aging. Even more, an article published in April of 2021 in the journal Aging found that following dietary recommendations (similar to the ones in this book) along with certain lifestyle modifications (like sleeping 7 hours/night, exercising 30 minutes 5 days/week, practicing breathing exercises 2x/day and taking high quality supplements) actually REVERSED AGING by 3 years in only 8 weeks time[7]. This research is mind-blowing. Albeit the study was done on a small population of men, the data is significant. I want you to take a moment and really take this in- **there is now scientific evidence showing that when you manage inflammation in your body you can reverse (or at least, slow down) the aging process.** I know for many women on the

#TTC path, the idea that they could be physiologically 3 years younger in this process would be so relieving.

If you want to take an even deeper dive into this topic of diet, lifestyle and aging, head to AimeeRaupp.com/EQDiet and watch the interview between Dr. Zaher Merhi (he's a reproductive endocrinologist I regularly work with) and I where we discuss this in greater detail.

Your takeaway here should be: **When I manage the inflammation in my body, I can improve the quality of my eggs, improve my cellular health *and* take a few years off of my genetic age.**

Why Is This Diet 100 Days Long?

Before I explain even more about inflammation and its impact on your aging ovaries, I want to address another important piece of this diet: how long it is. Many of you may be wondering, "Why is this diet 100 days long?"

It's because the process of folliculogenesis--which is the developmental process of your dormant ovarian follicles growing and maturing into a dominant follicle that your body will ovulate--typically takes 100 days. Based on that understanding of folliculogenesis and what medical research has shown, during those 100 days you can influence the health and vitality of your developing follicles.

According to a medical research article entitled, Nutritional Influences on Folliculogenesis, "folliculogenesis begins with a primordial follicle progressing into more developed stages (i.e. primary, secondary, pre-antral, and antral) in a continuous, progressive process to either ovulation or, as in most cases, to atresia. Even early stages of follicular formation and subsequent development are influenced by both internal (e.g. genotype) and/or external environmental (e.g. nutrition and environmental) factors. Among these external factors, nutrition is one of the most important affecting reproductive function. A number of studies have now shown that nutrition can have both positive and negative effects on follicular growth, oestrous activity, oocyte quality, blastocyst development, and pregnancy outcome. Therefore, understanding the intricate processes involved during folliculogenesis and the ways in which factors, such as nutrition, affect them is leading to new opportunities to improve pregnancy rates by influencing follicle development and oocyte quality[8]." The research for this article was conducted, like many research studies are, on animal models as they are easier to study in comparison to human models. But the data is clear-- nutrition impacts egg quality.

In fact, the case for nutrition and fertility has been studied for over a decade finding the same thing over and over-- a diet high in antioxidants, protein and good quality fats (like omega 3 fatty acids) and one low in processed, packaged, poor quality fats (like omega 6 fatty acids), pesticide-ridden foods is the way to go for balanced hormones and optimal fertility. The Harvard Nurses study, one of the largest human trials on how diet impacts fertility showed that women who ate a diet rich in vegetables and fruits (i.e. antioxidants) had more regular ovulations in comparison to women who did not. And that women who consumed the highest amount of monounsaturated fats (specifically in the form of avocados) during the IVF cycle were 3 times more likely to be successful in conceiving a child. The Harvard study also showed that men who ate a diet high in fruits and vegetables had better sperm[9]. Research from the *Journal of American Medical Association* (JAMA) revealed that women who ate non-organic diets (and thus consumed more pesticides) had fewer pregnancies and live births[10]. A publication from the journal *Aging Cell*, demonstrated that, "the lifelong consumption of a diet rich in omega-3 fatty acids prolongs reproductive function into advanced maternal age, while a diet rich in omega-6 fatty acids is associated with very poor reproductive success at advanced maternal age.[11] Did you catch that--**a diet rich in omega-3 fatty acid prolongs reproductive function into advanced maternal age.** A literature review conducted by Braverman Reproductive Immunology concluded that an increased omega-3 intake prior to conception was shown to positively impact embryo morphology in a study on women undergoing IVF cycle, promotes vascular development in the endometrium, reduces the risk of miscarriage, increases uterine blood flow, increase the length of pregnancy and reduce preterm birth and reduces placental inflammation when taking during the first trimester and through the pregnancy[12]. Said another way, you can improve the quality of your eggs, the inflammation in your body and how your reproductive system works when you follow *The Egg Quality Diet*.

So you see, if you take 100 days (or more) to get a handle on the inflammation in your body and manage any co-existing health challenges that may be impacting your fertility, you can turn things around *and* improve your egg quality. With this book, you are getting the exact dietary steps to take to maximize your egg quality and ovarian health, even in your 40's. This is the ultimate nutrition plan for getting the best eggs out of your ovaries and creating the best babies from them. Even more, if you're in a heterosexual partnership, it's a great plan to optimize sperm quality too.

How Inflammation Impacts
Your Health and Your Fertility

I want you to understand the massive role inflammation has on your overall health and fertility because I know, from my work with thousands of women, that knowledge will empower you to stick to *The Egg Quality Diet* plan. In 2017 I wrote my fourth book, *Body Belief: How To Heal Autoimmune Diseases, Radically Shift Your Health and Learn to Love Your Body More.* As the title depicts, this book is all about inflammation, the emotional and physical kind, and how it impacts autoimmune conditions. I wrote *Body Belief* a few years after my book *Yes, You Can Get Pregnant* was released as my clinical experience, and academic research led me to connect the dots between fertility challenges, inflammation, and autoimmunity.

Let me break it down for you.

I interact with thousands of women (literally tens of thousands of women like you each week via my social media channels and website) and I always get the question: "Why this diet?" Or I receive feedback like, "Isn't meat bad for fertility?" Or, "My friend went vegan and she got pregnant." Or, "My friend ate only pineapples and rice and she got pregnant." Or, "My friend read *Yes, You Can Get Pregnant* and it worked for her but it hasn't worked for me. What am I doing wrong?" I want to remind you that you aren't doing anything wrong, you just haven't found your personal recipe for success yet. *The Egg Quality Diet* (and its accompanying resource on AimeeRaupp.com/EQDiet) will help you figure out what works (and doesn't work) for you from a dietary perspective. Plus it'll give you an easy-to-follow framework.

But to be clear, the reason this diet works is because it's a well-formulated, clinically tested, elimination diet that has been shown (repeatedly through hundreds of different women's lab results) to reduce inflammation. And, as you learned from the research presented earlier in this book-- when inflammation is reduced, oxidation is reduced, mitochondrial function improves and cellular aging is delayed or potentially even reversed. The key to this diet plan is consistency and frequency. Yes, you can mess it up and it can still work but it will not work if you follow it for three or four weeks and then throw in the towel. I want you to invest the time and energy and resources this diet requires because it will help you on your path to motherhood.

The best part of an elimination diet is that you get to reintroduce the foods you remove and you get to decide (based on how your body reacts or doesn't) whether or not that food works for you. From there you develop your very own plan for success. I will lay out for you how to reintroduce foods and when (so follow my guidance there) and you will gain clarity and insight into your body and how it speaks to you through its symptoms.

How do you know if inflammation or autoimmunity is impacting your fertility? It's hard to say with certainty without my knowing your exact case, but what I have found is that it is likely if you have experienced one or more of the following issues (there's also a detailed questionnaire I give you on the next page to help you clarify how inflammation is impacting your health and fertility):

- Have been trying to conceive for 2 or more years without success
- Have had more than one miscarriage without a live birth in between
- Have a diagnosed autoimmune condition (like Hashimoto's, colitis, rheumatoid arthritis, or celiac sprue)
- Have been diagnosed with endometriosis, PCOS, or POI

- Have one or more copies of the MTHFR genetic mutation (you can read more about this mutation and how to test for it on AimeeRaupp.com)
- Have the COMT and/or Il-6 and/or FADS genetic mutation (you can test for all of these with genetic tests like 23 and me)
- Have had repeated failed IVF's, even with genetically tested embryos
- Can't seem to get any genetically normal embryos or your embryos don't mature to the blastocyst stage when doing IVF's.

Why? Because there is more at play in those cases than just fertility challenges. From my experience and research, I estimate that 60-70% of women dealing with fertility challenges are also dealing with an inflammatory and/or autoimmune condition as well.

Yes, upwards of 60-70% of women who are having difficulty conceiving have other medical factors, like endometriosis, recurrent pregnancy loss (RPL), PCOS, POI, endometritis, Hashimoto's, celiac sprue and colitis, at play that are compromising their bodies ability to get and stay pregnant. These conditions and the systemic, whole-body inflammation associated with them *need* to be addressed first otherwise the body will have a hard time prioritizing fertility. That's where *The Egg Quality Diet* comes in. *The Egg Quality Diet*, which is based upon the Autoimmune Paleo Diet (AIP) mixed with Chinese Medicine nutrition (which I have a master's of science in) and specific anti-inflammatory, fertility-enhancing foods will help you get to the root of the inflammation in your body, heal your gut and manage any coexisting medical issues that are in the way of your fertility.

An excerpt from my book, Yes, You Can Get Pregnant on the topic of the immune system and how it impacts fertility:

"A 2021 review of current research on this topic (immune system issues and fertility) was published in the journal Clinical, and Developmental Immunology concluded the following, "Autoimmune mechanism, as well as an increased productions of multiple autoantibodies, are involved in such infertility disorders as POF (now called POI), endometriosis, PCOS, unexplained infertility and repeatedly unsuccessful IVF attempts and may be responsible for the pathophysiology of preeclampsia or spontaneous abortions (miscarriages)." Said another way: research is showing that autoimmune mechanisms are playing a role in the most common fertility issues women are facing."[13]

If you're suddenly feeling worried about having a medical condition on top of fertility challenges, know that I am here to guide you through it and that it is manageable. It is my area of expertise and I assure you it is absolutely figureoutable (and if you head to AimeeRaupp.com/EQDiet I have a list of blood tests you can ask your doctor to do to see the level of inflammation and possible autoimmunity in your body). One of the tools I use to help women decipher if inflammation or autoimmunity are at play in their body is my Kink's In Your Body Questionnaire. Let's pause for a moment while you get out a pen and take tally of any of the symptoms you are currently experiencing as listed out here (please note: this questionnaire is also available for download on AimeeRaupp.com/EQDiet)

Kinks In Your Body Questionnaire

Take a few minutes and look through this list of signs & symptoms and check off anything you're currently experiencing on a regular basis (meaning 1 or more times a week); *if you only experience one of these signs/symptoms once every two weeks or once every month, don't check them.* Be honest and really reflect - just because some of these symptoms are common doesn't mean they're normal. Many of these symptoms are indicators of excess inflammation and possible autoimmunity in your body. Again, don't stress too much as the diet laid out in this book will help you manage excess inflammation and possible autoimmunity.

Check in once every week and track your continued progress.

- ☐ Acne
- ☐ Allergies
- ☐ Anemia
- ☐ Anxiety
- ☐ Asthma
- ☐ Blurred vision
- ☐ Bloating
- ☐ Body rashes
- ☐ Brain fog

☐ Bruise easily
☐ Chest congestion
☐ Colds (get them every time they go around the office)
☐ Cold hands and/or feet
☐ Cold sores
☐ Constipation
☐ Dark circles under your eyes
☐ Depression
☐ Dermatitis
☐ Diarrhea
☐ Difficulty concentrating
☐ Difficulty getting to or staying asleep
☐ Dizziness
☐ Dry hair
☐ Dry mouth
☐ Dry, brittle nails
☐ Dry skin
☐ Easy weight changes (up or down)
☐ Eating compulsively
☐ Eczema
☐ Excessive nasal mucus
☐ Faintness
☐ Fatigue
☐ Feeling groggy after a full night's sleep
☐ Floaters in the eye
☐ Frequent throat clearing
☐ Gas
☐ General feeling of malaise of weakness
☐ Hair thinning
☐ Headaches
☐ Heart palpitations
☐ Hives
☐ Hot flashes
☐ Hyperactivity

- ☐ Intense PMS
- ☐ Irritability
- ☐ Itchy ears
- ☐ Itchy, watery eyes
- ☐ Joint pain
- ☐ Joint stiffness
- ☐ Joint swelling
- ☐ Loss of appetite
- ☐ Mood swings
- ☐ Multiple miscarriages without a live birth in between
- ☐ Muscle pain
- ☐ Muscle stiffness
- ☐ Nasal congestion
- ☐ Nervousness
- ☐ Peeling nails
- ☐ Persistent cough
- ☐ Psoriasis
- ☐ Red bumps on face
- ☐ Red flaky skin
- ☐ Reflux
- ☐ Retaining water
- ☐ Rosacea
- ☐ Runny nose
- ☐ Shiny skin on hands & forearms
- ☐ Shortness of breath
- ☐ Sneezing frequently
- ☐ Sore throat
- ☐ Speech issues (slurring or stuttering)
- ☐ Sweat easily
- ☐ Swollen ankles
- ☐ Swollen eyes
- ☐ Swollen lips
- ☐ Thick, red, scaly patches on skin
- ☐ Thirsty, excessively

☐ Thyroid issues (previously diagnosed)
☐ Trouble breathing
☐ Trouble remembering things
☐ Trouble with balance and coordination
☐ Yellowing on the skin and/or whites of the eyes

As you go through each phase of *The Egg Quality Diet*, I highly encourage you to, once each week, fill out the Kinks In Your Body questionnaire so you can track the progress your body is making (I made a downloadable PDF of this questionnaire and it's available to you on AimeeRaupp.com/EQDiet). If any of this feels overwhelming, please remember: I am here to guide you each step of the way. As is the highly informative resources page I created for you at AimeeRaupp.com/EQDiet One thing I am very well known for saying is: your fertility is an extension of your health. So tracking your symptoms is a great way to see your health improve as you follow *The Egg Quality Diet*.

Why An Elimination Diet Is So Important For Addressing Inflammation

A lot of my clients come to me having already worked with a healthcare practitioner who has done some kind of food allergy test or panel and the first thing they want to tell me is, "Oh, I don't have any issues with X (insert any kind of food), my doctor did a food allergy test on me." And, I'm here to tell you, plain and simple: those food allergy tests are highly inaccurate. The only absolute way to know what your body can and cannot tolerate is by doing an elimination diet. If you want to take a deeper dive into why these food allergy tests are unreliable, head over to AimeeRaupp.com/EQDiet and check out the resources on that page covering this topic.

The bottom line: if you are dealing with a handful of kinks from the questionnaire above, have been having difficulty trying to get or stay pregnant and feel like your body needs a reset, an elimination diet is the next logical step for you. Not only does an elimination diet give you a ton of insight into your body and how it responds to the food you feed it, but it also gives your digestive system (aka your gut) time to heal. As I discuss in-depth in my book, *Body Belief,* optimizing your gut health is the most important piece to restoring proper immune function in your body and reducing inflammation. Said another way: optimizing your fertility has a lot to do with healing your gut. An elimination diet as laid out in this book will not only reduce inflammation, it will begin the gut healing process and allow your body to start absorbing all of it's nutrition properly. This will in turn allow all the cells in your body, including the ones that make up the eggs in your ovaries, to heal, thrive and turn back time.

Some of you may be wondering, "What if I don't have a lot of symptoms of inflammation, is this still the right diet for me?" This is a great question, and the answer is: if you've been having a hard time getting or staying pregnant and/or having unsuccessful fertility treatments (especially in regards to embryos fertilizing and growing healthily when doing IVF) then YES, you need to do this diet. As a lot of times, especially in women under the age of 40, the inflammation or immune issues may not show up as outward symptoms just yet but they could still be impacting your internal system (especially in cases like silent endometriosis or premature ovarian aging/insufficiency). And, no matter what, this way of eating is only going to optimize your ability to get and stay pregnant so you have nothing to lose by trying it.

Following *The Egg Quality Diet* as laid out herein will do so many things to benefit your health and fertility by reducing your exposure to toxins in your food while at the same time healing your gut so you can absorb all the nutrition your body requires to fully thrive.

One More Important Focus Of This Diet: Macronutrients

In addition to reducing inflammation, regulating your immune system, balancing your hormones, and healing your gut-- you need to be eating the correct macronutrients for your fertility. Macronutrients (or macros for short) are the three categories of nutrients you eat the most and provide you with what your body needs to optimally function: protein, carbohydrates, and fats. So when you're counting your macros, you're counting the grams of proteins, carbs, or fat that you're consuming. Don't worry you don't have to spend time each day calculating your macros, as I've already done that for you with this diet plan (but if you want to track them on your own, I highly recommend using the app MyFitnessPal). The reason I am bringing up the macro conversation is that I want you to understand what these macros are and how balancing them is so imperative to optimal fertility and egg quality. Scientists have discovered different macronutrient percentages for different health conditions. For instance, people dealing with cancer need a lot more fat than any other macronutrient as ketogenic diets have been shown to work best for them. When it comes to fertility, women who are trying to conceive seem to be most fertile with a macronutrient breakdown of 45% fat, 30% protein, and 25% carbs. Some data suggests that eating even more fat (where fat makes up

60% of your macros and a tad fewer carbs and protein)[14] is even more ideal, but i find that hard for my clients to maintain, especially while still maintaining the other macros. Dr. Jeffrey Russel of the Delaware Institute for Reproductive Medicine discovered something fascinating in his own clinical practice: shifting his patients from eating a diet that was nearly 60% carbs, 10% protein, 30% fat to a diet that was 25% carbs, 30% protein and 45% fat dramatically improved fertility. Many of the women who were following the diet of 60% carbohydrates were having continued IVF failures and not making any blastocysts. When their diet shifted to 25% carbs, 30% protein and 45% fat **they had four times the pregnancy success rate[15].** Although Dr Russel's study was conducted on a small group of women in his clinical practice, I have seen very similar results in my experience. Even more, the type of carbs, protein and fat you consume is extremely important-- you need to consume foods that are nutrient dense, antioxidant rich and minimally processed.

Remember: I am advocating for this way of eating because I have seen some major fertility shifts for clients of mine when following *The Egg Quality Diet*. One client finally cut out her favorite green lentil dish and her joint pain, migraines and loose bowel movements went away. Plus she got naturally pregnant (for the first time ever) after 8 years of trying to conceive and 23 failed assisted reproductive techniques. Another client finally got her macros right (after years of following other fertility diets) lost 40 pounds, her chronic eczema cleared up, her daily anxiety settled and she finally got pregnant with a healthy baby boy with an IUI (9 IUI's previous to the diet all failed). One woman started the diet with her FSH at a 60 and by three months into the diet, her FSH was a 12. Dozens of women who switched from the general fertility diets out there to *The Egg Quality Diet* went from never making any blastocysts or genetically normal embryos to making them. For all my Stories of Hope, head to the resources page we have set up for you (AimeeRaupp.com/EQDiet) and hear all the details on what worked for women just like you.

It is my hope that by now you are armed with the reasons why this diet works. Now, the next step is diving into *The Egg Quality Diet* plan so we can turn around your fertility journey and get you pregnant.

CHAPTER TWO

The Basics of *The Egg Quality Diet* Plan

As I have mentioned already, *The Egg Quality Diet* is an elimination diet. Let's break down how it works. First, you will begin this diet in **Phase One** where, over a 9-day period, you will begin to remove the foods that have been found to be inflammatory, nutrient-poor, and triggering to autoimmunity and therefore do not support your health or your fertility. Then in **Phase Two,** you will be eating a very balanced and nutrient-dense, although limited diet, for 11 days. In **Phase Three**, which lasts 4 weeks, you get to add in some of the foods you eliminated. And finally, in **Phase Four**, which lasts 8 weeks, you start reintroducing more foods until you find exactly what works (and doesn't work) for your body. You remain in Phase Four for a minimum of 8 weeks but you can thrive here for however long you'd like. And, as I said, at the beginning of each week of the diet you will revisit the kinks in your body questionnaire (there's a downloadable version of this questionnaire at AimeeRaupp.com/EQDiet so you can easily print off several copies) and make note of how the inflammation in your body is shifting. Also as you get deeper into this program and get the diet piece down pat, I will start layering in some important lifestyle recommendations to help you maximize this protocol and get pregnant faster. So be certain to read through all the phases as they are laid out in this book as I layer in a lot of information that will help you get and stay pregnant.

One thing that is important to note before you dive in is that in a few cases, some women following this diet began experiencing more digestive issues, like increased bloating or gas or reflux, than is common (as most women doing this diet feel major improvements in their digestive health; however if you don'tf, please head to the resources section in this book (on page 229) and read about how histamines and/or a condition called small intestine bacterial overgrowth (SIBO) could be at play and what to do about it. Additionally, if you know you have histamine issues or have been diagnosed with SIBO, you should also head to the resources section and follow my direction on how to do this diet keeping those conditions in mind.

First Things First

As I discuss in my other books, especially *Yes, You Can Get Pregnant*, for optimal fertility and egg quality you need to be eating plenty of organic, non-genetically modified foods such as pastured eggs, grass-fed meats (including organ meats), free-range chicken, wild fish, gelatinous rich bone broths and a ton of cooked, organic vegetables. But before I dive into all the specifics, I want to ask you to take a deep breath and read the following section two or three times (I bolded it for you intentionally).

These dietary changes may all seem like a lot, so let me remind you of two things:

1. **You are cutting out these foods because they can all be highly inflammatory, disruptive to gut health, and triggering autoimmunity** *all of which can be impacting your fertility and egg quality.*
2. **As I explained, this is an elimination diet which means after you eliminate the foods for a set period of time you can reintroduce the foods you miss the most and see how you react based on the kinks in your body questionnaire. But know this, some foods (like the highly processed ones) I will urge you to never reintroduce.**

3. **Let me say that last bit again: YOU AREN'T ELIMIN.. THESE FOODS FOREVER. You can reintroduce them and see how you feel and create a style of eating that best supports your body.**

If you want to understand the in-depth reasons on the why behind cutting out all these foods I encourage you to read my book *Body Belief* and the book, *The Paleo Approach* by Sarah Ballantyne. In a nutshell, all of the foods we are to eliminate during this program contain low-level toxic substances (like lectins and saponins) that increase intestinal permeability and cause inflammation in your body. But not every person's body will react the same way to the same foods, hence why we remove them and then reintroduce them. Look at it like this: you are not just removing certain foods but rather you are adding in more nutrient-dense foods that your body can better utilize so it can thrive.

Some Words On Nourishing You

I know you are gearing up to dive into this diet but because I've been doing the work I do for almost 20 years, I need to say a few more words to you…

I know you picked up this book because you are looking for help conceiving. This book will do that and more; it will help you improve your health nutritionally (and the resources found in my other books and at AimeeRaupp.com/EQDiet will help you optimize your health beyond nutrition) so that you can see your body transform, regain hope and optimize your health and fertility. But I also want to tell you that the diet laid out in this book is much more than that. The food you choose to nourish your body with creates the internal environment in which every single bodily process occurs. So you see, this is about so much more than egg quality or balanced hormones… this is about you transforming yourself. I know you just want to get pregnant but I really want it to be more than that for you.

Here's what I wish for you to gain from this way of eating:

- I want this baby of yours to grow and develop in the healthiest environment possible so that it can get all it needs to thrive in our world.
- I want your body to have all the nutrition it needs so that it can grow a human (which is a really important job) but also have a strong pregnancy and a seamless postpartum recovery.
- I want you to have plenty of breastmilk if you decide to breastfeed your child.
- I want you to be healthy enough to go on to have another child if you so desire.
- I want your body to have less inflammation because that means you will be less likely to experience inflammatory conditions like heart disease, type II diabetes, arthritis, Alzheimer's, and cancer as you age.
- I want you to do this diet and let yourself feel how good it is to feel good because you deserve that.

I know you will do it in the beginning because you just want to get to your baby as fast as you can, and I absolutely respect that. But I hope you continue eating this way for years to come because it has transformed your body and its trillions of cells.

Finding Peace On This Diet

One of my most influential spiritual teachers, Abraham Hicks, has said, "If you make peace with everything that you eat - no matter what it is- you'll thrive." I share this because I know you are human and that following this eating plan may have its challenges. I am asking you to be easy on yourself if you have moments where you fall off the plan. I would much rather you fall off the plan and enjoy whatever it is you decide to eat *and enjoy every single bite of it*. What I want you to avoid is falling off the plan and beating yourself up over it. There's an entire other premise to my work that I label emotional inflammation (which you can learn more about it on AimeeRaupp.com/EQDiet) but basically, your thoughts, especially the abusive ones, can be very inflammatory to your body and its cells. What I am trying to say is: following this diet and then falling off the plan, and then beating yourself up over it, and then doing that repeatedly, is not going to be of help to your health or your fertility. I'd much rather you meet yourself with compassion and kindness and find peace while following this plan. Many of my clients tell me this way of eating has changed their life and they will never go back to their old ways. I would love that for you too.

Picture it: you are thoughtfully food shopping for quality ingredients that you are excited to cook with. You are preparing your meal with love and appreciation for the nourishment it will provide. You are then eating and sharing your meal with others all with a grateful heart. If this sounds somewhat unrealistic to you, don't worry, in the pages that follow, I provide you with all the tools to make this shift as simple and doable as possible. The key is being mindful and viewing food as so much more than something we eat, but something that enhances our health, something that comes from nature to provide our bodies with nutrients for optimal functioning, and most importantly a tool you can use to not only improve your fertility and egg quality but your life emotionally and spiritually. When you view cooking and eating as an extension of your health you will increase your odds of getting pregnant.

It is my hope that my pregnancies in my 40's, and the pregnancies of the thousand's of my patients who have followed this approach, serve as inspiration to all of you to really apply all that I talk about in this book (and in my books: *Yes, You Can Get Pregnant* and *Body Belief*). It is my hope that the stories of women who have gone before you will motivate you to take back control over your health by vigilantly embracing the nutritional approach I have laid out herein. It is my hope that you no longer live in fear over what your doctors have told you or what you have read on the internet about your fertility. It is my hope that you put an end to letting your fertility challenges define you. Rather, I hope you embrace the fact that your health and fertility are in your hands. You can improve your fertility, you are not broken, your body is dynamic and smart and it innately knows how to conceive. Dig into this book, make use of all the resources I created for you on AimeeRaupp.com/EQDiet, restore some hope in your heart and get on track with reminding your female reproductive system of what it inherently knows how to do—create genetically normal eggs, conceive and carry to term a healthy baby. You really do have the power to change your health and improve your fertility. With that said, I need to ask this of you: can you try—*just try*—to believe in your fertility more than you don't? That will really set us off on a positive trajectory that will massively influence your ability to optimize your health and fertility.

OK, take a deep breath, thank yourself for beginning to have hope again, and join me on this nutritional journey that will optimize your health and fertility while cultivating a more grateful heart and home for you and your family. Now, let's get into what you can eat and what you are going to eliminate on this diet.

There Are So Many Possibilities When You're Open To Trying New Things

The fact that you are still here tells me that you are ready for change and you are open to new possibilities. So let's get right to it.

As I have stated, *The Egg Quality Diet* follows the same basic parameters as the diet I laid out in *Yes, You Can Get Pregnant*, which means you are to avoid, what I call: The 6 Big No's:

Gluten
Pesticides
Artificial Sweeteners
Soy
Genetically Modified Foods
Added Sugars

Plus this diet cuts out dairy too. In *Yes, You Can Get Pregnant* I did allow organic, full-fat dairy in moderation (a few ounces, a few times a week) however since writing that book I have realized that many women do better completely off dairy, especially if they have inflammatory, gut, hormonal or autoimmune issues.

You will also see, as part of the elimination diet we also cut out the potentially inflammatory foods below. Generally speaking the foods we are focused on cutting out or eliminating have been scientifically shown to contribute to gut dysbiosis, autoimmunity, inflammatory diseases, tissue degeneration (like the important fertile tissue in your ovaries and uterus) are typically highly processed, filled with pesticides, and molds and for many, are very difficult to digest. For a breakdown as to why we are eliminating the below foods, check out the videos I have on AimeeRaupp.com/EQDiet on this topic, as well my book *Body Belief* and the book, *The Paleo Approach* by Sarah Ballantyne go into great detail on this topic):

> Legumes
> Nightshade vegetables
> Grains and pseudograins
> Processed vegetable oils
> Nuts and seeds
> Egg whites
> Coffee and alcohol

Before you continue reading, take a deep breath and remember: these eliminations aren't forever. We are eliminating all of these foods to give your body a break from them, so you can decipher how they are impacting your body and so you can give yourself a much needed fertility reboot. And, there's still A LOT of food that you can eat (I have it all mapped out for you!)

For your ease, on the pages that follow you will see a handful of amazing reference material that I created to help you best succeed on *The Egg Quality Eating Plan.* You will see:

- The Egg Quality Diet Guide (which is a breakdown of what you can and can't eat during each phase of this plan)
- An extensive list of what I have found to be the best anti-aging, fertility enhancing, egg quality boosting foods
- Hack sheets for bone broth, fertility, liver support soup (a key part of this diet), and fat bombs
- And, a guide to all the culinary seasonings you can use broken up by Phases of this eating plan

Keep in mind, I also put all of this material on AimeeRaupp.com/ EQDiet, I urge you to head there now to download and print out these materials and put them in a folder or hang them on your refrigerator or somewhere you can easily access them.

THE EGG QUALITY DIET GUIDE

This 'cheat sheet' (which is also available to download on AimeeRaupp.com/EQDiet) is to help you navigate which foods you can eat during each Phase of the Egg Quality Diet. This is an elimination diet and we will be cutting out ALL of the following foods (**TO BE CLEAR**, you will begin removing these foods in the Phase 1 Phase; completely remove them in Phase 2; begin reintroducing them *as instructed later in this book* in Phases 3 and 4):

Gluten

Soy

Dairy

Nuts

Beans

Grains (including corn flours)

Pseudograins

Artificial sweeteners

Added sugar

Nightshade vegetables

Egg whites

Refined vegetable oils

Fruit (only in Phase 2)

Alcohol

Coffee

Certain spices & seasonings *(see below chart for specifics)*

To successfully heal your body and your gut, it is imperative that you take a break from ALL of the above foods for a certain period of time (as instructed); In their place, you will be eating many delicious and nutrient-dense foods. Enjoy!

Food Group	Phase 1	Phase 2	Phase 3 &4	Avoid Always
Dairy	Start cutting back; ideally limit to one serving daily of an organic, full-fat dairy product.	No dairy at all, replace with: Coconut milk (full fat or lite) Ghee Coconut milk yogurt Coconut kefir	Reintroduce FERMENTED dairy products as directed later on in the book. Grass-fed butter Full fat fermented yogurt, kefir, butter Raw cheese. If you have a diagnosed autoimmune condition, you should avoid dairy (with the exception of ghee, which is technically	Low fat, non-organic milk, cheese, cottage cheese, cream, yogurt, butter, ice cream, non-dairy creamers

			dairy-free butter) now and forever.	
Gluten, Grains & Pseudograin s (& corn)	Start cutting back	No gluten, grains, or pseudograin s. Replace with: Sweet potato 'toast' Kale chips Parsnip chips Zoodles Cauliflower fried rice Sweet Potato fries (see recipe section at the back of this book)	Once you reintroduce fruit in Phase 3, you can have plantain chips. Reintroduce non-gluten grains & pseudograin s as directed later on in the book. Soaked, organic rice and quinoa Reintroduce gluten-free flours at week twelve: blanched almond flour, coconut flour, arrowroot powder, and tapioca starch Reintroduce non-GMO	All non-organic gluten-containing foods. Non-organic corn and corn flours. It is ideal that you avoid gluten for the rest of your life however, after twelve weeks on this plan AND all of your symptoms have dramatically improved, you can try some fermented or sprouted ORGANIC glutinous grains and see how you react. If you have a diagnosed

			and organic corn as directed later on in the book.	autoimmune condition, you should avoid gluten now and forever.
Nuts and Seeds	Start cutting back. And focus on only consuming organic and sprouted nuts and seeds	No nuts or seeds. Replace with: Avocado Egg yolk Bone Broth Fish Roe Vegetables Approved oils & fats	Reintroduce SOAKED and/or SPROUTED nuts and seeds as directed later on in the book.	All nuts and seeds that are not organic and raw. You should only consume sprouted and or soaked nuts and seeds. NO PEANUTS ever as they are filled with mold and enterotoxins both of which are highly inflammatory.
Vegetables	Eat a lot of them. Switch to organic and begin avoiding nightshades.	Eat only the following vegetables in Phase 2: Spinach, kale, broccoli, butternut squash,	Reintroduce all vegetables except nightshades. Again, be sure you eat more cooked than raw vegetables.	Non-organic corn, creamed vegetables, canned vegetables.

		dandelion greens, sweet potato, asparagus, cauliflower, sea vegetables or beets. Consume mainly steamed, sauteed or roasted. You can have some raw veggies, but most of your vegetables should be cooked. I like the 80/20 rule (80% cooked, 20% raw).	In phase 4 of this plan, you can try reintroducin g nightshade vegetables as directed later on in the book.	
Legumes (Beans)	Start cutting back. And focus on only consuming organic and sprouted beans	No legumes (beans). Replace with: Avocado Egg yolk Bone Broth Fish Roe Vegetables Approved oils & fats	Reintroduce SOAKED and/or SPROUTED legumes (beans) as directed in Phase 4 of this plan. Keep in mind cacao and carob are in the	All legumes (beans) that are not organic and raw. You should only consume sprouted and or soaked nuts and seeds. NO PEANUTS.

			legume (bean) family. So, you can also add back in raw chocolate when you add legumes back in!	
Eggs	Enjoy. But be sure you are buying organic eggs from pastured chickens.	You can eat only egg yolks from pastured organic chickens during Phase 2	Reintroduce the entire egg from pastured organic chickens as directed in Phase 4 of this plan	Conventional, non-organic eggs.
Protein	Enjoy grass-fed, pastured animal products and wild-caught fish (follow Monterey Bay Aquarium rec's: https://www.seafoodwatch.org/recommendations/download-consumer-guides	Grass-fed beef or lamb or wild-caught salmon or cod	Enjoy grass-fed, pastured animal products and wild-caught fish	Commercially/factory-raised animal products, commercially/factory-farmed fish products

Fruit	Enjoy all organic fruits.	Only avocados, lemons, and limes	Enjoy fruit again! Have 6-8 servings per week of low sugared fruits (melons, berries, grapefruit, and avocado) Have 2-4 servings per week of moderate-to-high-sugared fruits: apples, apricots, kiwi, nectarine, papaya, plum, pomegranate, pears, plum, peach, citrus (all others except grapefruit), banana, mango, pineapple, plantains, watermelon, dates, and fresh figs.	Non-organic fruits, fruit in a can, processed fruit juices. Have dried fruits and 100% pure fruit juices (not from concentrate) very sparingly, like once/month max.

Oils and Fats	Begin reading labels and avoiding all processed and refined vegetable oils	Consume extra virgin, cold-pressed olive oil, avocado oil, coconut oil, palm oil, lard, tallow, ghee & the 'Happy Egg Mayo' from the recipes section	Consume extra virgin, cold-pressed olive oil, avocado oil, coconut oil, palm oil, lard, tallow, ghee & the 'Happy Egg Mayo' from the recipes section Reintroduce grass-fed butter in Phase 4 of this book as directed	Butter, margarine, shortening, soybean oil, cottonseed oil, palm kernel oil, rapeseed oil, sunflower oil, corn oil, peanut oil, safflower oil, canola oil, and any mayonnaise or salad dressings (made with any of these ingredients)
Drinks	Start reading labels and cut out all drinks with added sugar. Focus on drinking filtered water, organic green tea, organic black tea, organic herbal teas, seltzer or mineral water, coconut	During Phase 2 there is no alcohol or coffee; limited organic black tea and green tea if needed.	Reintroduce coffee and alcohol in Phase 4 as directed later on in this book. Keep in mind, when you reintroduce them, you can have organic coffee & "Clean" alcoholic	Alcoholic beverages more than 5 drinks per week, non-organic coffee, soda pop, soft drinks

	water, kombuchas (stay with the ones that have under 5 grams of sugar)		drinks such as top-shelf vodka or tequila and/or organic wine in moderation and depending on how you react to it. AimeeRaupp .com/wine is the only Aimee Approved wine	
Sugars & Artificial Sweeteners	Try to limit added sugars and especially artificial sweeteners and sugars as discussed on pages 81-82 of Body Belief. If you really want sweeteners, use honey, maple syrup, stevia, or coconut sugar.	No sugars or sweeteners	Reintroduce honey, maple syrup, stevia, sugar in the raw or coconut sugar as directed in Phase 4 of this program.	Refined sugar, white/brow n sugars, high fructose corn syrup, agave, xylitol, evaporated cane juice, Splenda®, Equal®, Sweet'N Low®

Condiments, Spices & Seasonings	Begin cutting out all processed, sugar-filled condiments that contain any of the oils and fats that are not approved. As well, limit intake or remove completely of any spice/season ing that contains nightshade vegetables and/or curries.	During Phase 2 you are only to have the following spices & seasonings: Apple cider vinegar, lemon juice, lime juice, parsley, ginger, turmeric, cinnamon, cilantro, and good quality sea salt	In Phase 3& 4 you can use any of the spices and seasonings listed on page 58 In Phase 4 of the plan, you can try reintroducin g nightshade vegetable-based spices & seasonings (including curries). As directed in Phase 4 you can also add back in raw honey, maple syrup, and raw cacao powder.	Processed and non-organic condiments that contain toxic sugars (like high fructose corn syrup) and oils (like soy oil). Be sure to read ingredients of all condiments, spices, and seasonings, in particular: ketchup, relish, chutney, soy sauce, barbecue sauce, salad dressings, and teriyaki sauce.

Easy Egg Quality Diet Hacks

Instead of this:	Eat this:
Soy Sauce/Tamari	Coconut Aminos
Soda	Kombucha and/or sparkling water
Butter/Margarine	Cultured ghee
Splenda etc	Raw Honey, Raw sugar, Coconut sugar, Maple syrup & Stevia
Chocolate	Raw Cacao
Protein Powders	Collagen Peptides/Bone Broth Protein
Store Bought (non paleo Mayo)	Homemade mayo/ Paleo mayo's (Primal Kitchen brand)
Marinara sauce	No-mato sauce

Fertility Enhancing Foods

When it comes to fertility from a Traditional Chinese Medicine (TCM) perspective, we are all about keeping the uterus (aka The Child's Palace) warm and cozy. What that means is from a viewpoint, optimal fertility means you should be eating warm foods rather than cold, room temperature at a minimum; adopt an 80/20 rule of cooked/raw foods. For example, if eating fruit, take it out of the fridge a few hours before eating and leave them on the counter. Always be sure that all protein sources are grass-fed and organic, and, when looking at produce, use the Dirty Dozen and Clean 15 lists from EWG to help save money (see links in the resources section and on AimeeRaupp.com/EQDiet).

These are foods I've already worked into your meal plans and you'll want to continue eating regularly even after the program. Check out AimeeRaupp.com/EQDiet and the resources section in this book for links on where to purchase some of my favorite items on this diet.

- Bone broth
- Vital Proteins collagen peptides
- Meat (grass-fed and organic; we use ButcherBox.com for our home)
- Eggs (pasture-raised and organic)
- Fish (wild-caught unless where noted acceptable, see this link for more info:http://www.seafoodwatch.org/seafood-recommendations/consumer-guides)
- Liver and other organ meats (from grass-fed organic animals- or as a supplement)
- Fish roe (you can buy a good quality one from VitalChoice.com)
- Leafy greens
- Cruciferous veggies
- Broccoli sprouts
- Onions
- Root veggies

- Mushrooms
- Sweet potatoes and yams
- Fermented foods
- Avocado
- Turmeric
- Garlic
- Berries
- Stone fruit
- Green tea/matcha
- Coconut oil/coconut butter
- Ghee (be certain it's a certified dairy-free brand)

Additional Aimee Faves to Boost Your Fertility:

- Organic blackstrap molasses
- Royal jelly
- Cordyceps (can be taken as a supplement)
- Spirulina or blue-green algae (can be taken as a supplement)
- Black chicken (yes, there is such a thing)
- Sunflower seeds (depending on the your Phase in *The Egg Quality Diet*)
- Sesame seeds - especially black (depending on the your Phase in *The Egg Quality Diet*)
- Flax seeds (depending on the your Phase in *The Egg Quality Diet*)

- Pumpkin seeds (depending on the your Phase in *The Egg Quality Diet*)
- Chia seeds (depending on the your Phase in *The Egg Quality Diet*)
- Acai (depending on the your Phase in *The Egg Quality Diet*)

Bone Broth Hacks

Bone broth on its own is a savory liquid with health benefits to boot, but even the best broth can use some jazzing up now and then. Once you've done the work of slow simmering your bone broth (or purchasing the packaged ones I've recommended on AimeeRaupp.com/EQDiet and in the resources section), you can stir in any of these mix-ins, adding extra flavor and nutrients (be certain to make sure you are following the rules of whichever Phase of this eating plan you are in when adding the below to your broth).

Savory and Creamy
Stir mix-in of choice into bone broth; simmer for 15 minutes. Serve warm.

Creamy and Dreamy: 6 c. bone broth + 1 c. full fat coconut milk
Build Me Up Buttercup: 6 c. bone broth + 1 tbsp cultured ghee
Umami: 6 c. bone broth + 2 tbsp coconut aminos
I'll Avo'nother: 6 c. bone broth + 2 c. cubed avocado

Veggie Goodness
Stir mix-in of choice into bone broth; simmer for 20 minutes. Serve warm.

Kale Yeah! 6 c. bone broth + 2 c. chopped kale
Harvest: 6 c. bone broth + 1 c. butternut squash cubed
Shroomfest: 6 c. bone broth + 1 c. shiitake mushrooms
Cabbage Patch: 6 c. bone broth + 2 c. chopped cabbage
It's the Fennel Countdown: 6 c. bone broth + ? c. thinly sliced fennel
Jalapeño Business (after week 10 of Reawaken): 6 c. bone broth + ¼ c. sliced jalapeño
Bright & Tangy: 6 c. bone broth + 2 stalks lemongrass sliced
Under the Sea: 6 c. bone broth + sprinkle of dulse flakes or a few sheets of kelp sliced

Herbs and Spices
Stir mix-in of choice into bone broth; simmer for 15 minutes. Serve warm.

Thyme of Your Life:: 6 c. bone broth + 2 sprigs fresh thyme
Green Goodness: 6 c. bone broth + 2 tbsp chopped basil

Fertility Smoothie Guide

Call it a smoothie, call it a protein shake, a blended beverage by any other name is just as sweet (and nutrient-dense!). We aren't talking about something you get in the mall food court, though. Your smoothies are going to be SUPER low in sugar (even natural sugar) and made of delicious, nourishing whole foods. It may seem daunting at first but once you learn the basics you'll be whipping up your own recipes in a snap!

The Basics:

1. Protein: You're only going to be using clean protein with no fillers. Grab some Vital Proteins Collagen Peptides and some Ancient Nutrition Bone Broth Protein. You can use either or even a scoop of each.
2. Liquid: We're keeping it simple here, folks! Use either filtered water or full-fat coconut milk, or a combo of both depending on the consistency you're looking for. (Once you're reintroducing nuts you can use almond milk, macadamia nut milk, or cashew milk, just make sure you're watching for reactions and the ingredients as many store-bought nut milks contain a lot of sugar and not so clean ingredients.)
3. Greens: Don't make a smoothie without them! A handful (a cup) of steamed or blanched spinach or kale will do your body good (*we are not into too much cold or raw foods in The Egg Quality Diet plan because it can make your uterus cold and inhospitable*)

4. Fat: Fat will keep you full, work wonders for your skin, hair, and nails, and will fuel your body! Consider throwing in some coconut oil, ghee, or, for a super creamy smoothie, half an avocado.

5. Throw in one or more of your favorite fertility-enhancing foods (from the Fertility Enhancing Foods reference sheet)

6. Phase 3& 4 Bonus: Fruit: Grab some berries, a banana, an apple or pear, whatever low-sugared fruit suits your fancy, ¾ cup.

7. Add some flair: Throw in some ginger, cinnamon, mint, matcha, or lemon to jazz it up! (Once you've reintroduced beans in Phase 4 you can also throw in some cacao powder, again just watch for reactions).

8. Temperature: We aren't about too many cold or raw foods on *The Egg Quality Diet*. Wherever possible use room temp ingredients. If something needs to be refrigerated let it sit out on the counter for a bit before making your smoothie.

Smoothie Hacks:

1. Blanching your greens will make them even easier to digest.

2. Invest in a good blender. Not only will it make smoothies better, it'll be great for soups and sauces, even making your own mayo!

3. Have limited access to fresh fruit and veggies? Buy some bags of frozen and pull out a serving the night before so you don't have frozen in the morning. Or, when fruit and veggies are plentiful at the farmer's market, stock up and freeze until you're ready to use them.

4. Have spare mason jars? Make a big batch of smoothies and freeze them in individual servings. Again, put them in the fridge the night before and then, upon waking, put it on the counter to come to room temp.

5. Liquid first! This gives the blades room to move and makes a smoother smoothie.

Fat Bomb Hacks

What is a fat bomb?

Basically, fat bombs are a mix of fat and seasonings melted and mixed together. They are like fudge that is good for you. And, they are the perfect snack to get you through Phase 1 &2 of *The Egg Quality Diet*. Make them and snack on them (keeping it to one tablespoon serving daily). Be certain you are following the rules of whichever Phase of *The Egg Quality Diet* you are in when making these delicious bites below.

STEP ONE: Find your fat base
Fat bombs need fat that will solidify in the fridge and, ideally, stay solid at room temp (softening is fine)

PURIFY Phase approved fats for Fat Bombs:
Cultured Ghee
Coconut Oil
Coconut Butter
Coconut Milk (canned- the boxed milk-like kind won't solidify)

STEP TWO: Grab your spices/mix-ins
Phase 2 approved seasonings for Fat Bombs:
Coconut Meat/Shreds
Citrus
Cinnamon
Ginger
Turmeric
Sea Salt

STEP THREE: Put it all together
Melt your fat base and blend or mix in your desired ingredients. Then pour into a tray to cut into squares (after solidifying), pour into fun-shaped silicone molds (Jaymes loves his dinos and robots), or let cool slightly and roll into balls (definitely the hardest method of the three).

Once you're in Phase 3 & 4 and have successfully reintroduced foods you can start adding them to your fat bombs. Some yummy ideas include vanilla, berries, cacao powder, and nut butters.

That's it! It's a super simple way to get in much needed fat and help curb sugar cravings.

Liver Support Juice Hacks

A key part of Phases 2, 3 & 4 of *The Egg Quality Diet* is the liver support soup (recipe is below and also on p. X) and even though I love the recipe as is, not everyone does. So, my team and I have come up with a few hacks for you:

ORIGINAL RECIPE: LIVER SUPPORT SOUP

Yield: 3 to 4 servings

Ingredients
4 beets, cooked
3 carrots, blanched
1-inch piece fresh ginger, peeled and minced
4 to 6 pieces of fresh turmeric (or 1 heaping teaspoon ground turmeric)
1 large handful of cilantro, stems included
1 large handful of dandelion greens, stems included
1 large handful of parsley
Juice of 2 lemons
1/4 teaspoon freshly ground black pepper
1/4 teaspoon sea salt
1 garlic clove (or 1/4 teaspoon organic garlic powder for a milder flavor)
1 cup of bone broth
1/2 cup of filtered water

Directions

1. Blend all the ingredients; add 1/2 cup of filtered water if it's too thick for your liking. Enjoy! Makes 2 to 3 servings. Reserve additional servings, broken up into 6 to 8-ounce portions in the freezer, and thaw as needed.

Liver Support Soup Hack #1: Blend all the ingredients with an additional ½ cup of water, transfer the mixture to a stainless steel saucepan, heat up, and drink like a soup. Top with some avocado if you desire.

Liver Support Soup Hack #2: Blend all the ingredients with no bone broth and rather 2 cups of water and drink. If you water it down more, it will be easier to drink.

Liver Support Soup Hack #3: Blend all the ingredients with 2 cups of bone broth and a full bag of steamed spinach, transfer the mixture to a stainless steel saucepan, heat up, and drink like a soup. Top with some avocado if you desire. This is how I typically consume it, it's delicious!

Liver Support Soup Hack #4: This is for those of you who just can't consume this as a soup. Choose some of the ingredients in the recipe and find ways to add them to your meals throughout the day. For example, add extra beets to a meal or some cilantro. Cool with garlic and turmeric and ginger. Just focus on getting in these ingredients daily as they support liver detoxification in a major way.

Seasoning Guide

You're going to be cooking a LOT while following *The Egg Quality Diet* so here is a list of approved ways to spice up your food. Anything listed below can be used both dried or fresh but either way I highly recommend organic. **If you don't see something listed below then you shouldn't use it until you're in Phase 4 and have successfully begun reintroductions.**

- Basil
- Bay leaves
- Chamomile
- Chervil
- Chives
- Cilantro
- Cinnamon
- Cloves
- Dill
- Garlic
- Ginger
- Horseradish
- Lavender
- Lemon balm
- Mace
- Marjoram leaves
- Onion
- Oregano
- Parsley
- Peppermint
- Rosemary

- Saffron
- Sage
- Salt
- Savory
- Spearmint
- Tarragon
- Thyme
- turmeric

The following seasonings and spices may be used in moderation (1-2 times a week) in Phase 3.

- Allspice
- Black pepper
- Caraway
- Cardamom
- Green peppercorn
- Juniper
- Pink peppercorn
- Star anise
- Vanilla bean
- White pepper

On The Go Snack Ideas

I know how hectic life can be, so I went ahead and gathered some easy on-the-go snacks for you that can be store-bought. As of when I wrote this book (March 2021), these snacks and brands are all approved for *The Egg Quality Diet*, but always read ingredients to be certain:

Epic Cranberry Bison Bars

Organic Gemini Raw Tiger Nuts

Artisana Coconut Butter

Bare Simply Cinnamon Organic Apple Chips

Dang Lightly Salted Toasted Coconut Chips

Nutiva Coconut Manna

Jackson's Honest Sweet Potato Chips

Freeze Dried Blueberries

Sea Snax

Wild Planet Wild Alaskan Salmon

Wild Planet Sardines

Wild Planet Clams

Organic Apple Butter

Pork Clouds Rosemary & Sea Salt Pork Rinds

Paleo Angel Power Balls

Yucan Crunch

Wild Zora Lamb & Veggie Jerky

Pure Traditions Cranberry Beef & Organ Strips

Barnana Plantain Chips

Anita's Plain Coconut Milk Yogurt

GT's Kombucha

Trader Joe's Organic Coconut Smoothie

keep in mind you will likely be able to find all of these products on Amazon.com

Chapter Three

Phase 1 (9 days; week 1 & partial week 2)

OK, you are now armed with your reference guides and hack sheets *plus* all the reasons why this is the diet that can finally help you get and stay pregnant. Now, let's dive into Phase 1 of *The Egg Quality Diet*. This is the phase where we will eliminate all the foods mentioned so that we can begin to completely revamp your internal landscape for the better. Get prepared for an entire cellular overhaul!. In the pages that follow you will be given step-by-step guidance on how to start the first phase of this diet, which lasts 9 days. In this chapter, you will also have a menu all laid out for you. And, there are some great recipes in the back of this book for you along with weekly shopping lists which have been created based on the menu laid out herein. All of your shopping lists are also on AimeeRaupp.com/EQDiet where you can download them and print them out for ease when doing your weekly food shopping.

Phase 1 Menu

> *REMEMBER: This is just a template for you to use, you can continue to eat your foods of choice as long as you eliminate the recommended foodstuffs as directed for each day. Shopping lists for this phase (and all phases) are in the back of this book as well as available for download on AimeeRaupp.com.EQDiet. All the recipes you need are in the back of this book.*

Pointers for this phase of *The Egg Quality Diet*:

- This phase's mantra is: **I am open to the possibility of things working out for me.** Repeat this mantra to yourself often. Even better, write it out on a post-it and stick it where you will see it.
- You will begin reading labels and cut back (eventually, remove entirely) the foods that definitely do not support your healing process: added sugar, soy, refined vegetable oils, gluten, genetically modified (GM) foods, and more.
- Take a moment at the beginning of this week to honestly fill out your Kinks In Your Body Questionnaire (found on page 21 and also available for download at AimeeRaupp.com/ EQDiet)
- You will have FUN at the foodstore buying all of your favorite fertility healing foods (if you're like me and do your food shopping on Sundays, then print out this week's shopping list from AimeeRaupp.com/EQDiet and head to your grocery store!)
- You will clean out your kitchen and pantry and get rid of all the foods that don't support your health or fertility
- You will become reacquainted with your kitchen and begin cooking more
- If you have one, you will learn to nix that artificial sweetener and/or diet soda habit
- Keep the daily tips (listed below) in mind throughout the week
- And, most importantly, be easy on yourself (check out some of my meditations on AimeeRaupp.com/EQDiet to help with that).
- If you are already following most of the dietary recommendations covered in Phase 1, I recommend you use

this time to really fine-tune your diet and make sure you are truly eliminating everything recommended.

- For all those COLD TURKEY folks, if you just want to quit ALL the eliminated foods cold turkey, you are welcome to do so at any time before we begin Phase 2 on day 10. Just be aware that you can get some intense withdrawal symptoms from sugar, caffeine, and alcohol (depending on how much you regularly consume of each). So give yourself a few days off of those specific foodstuffs BEFORE you begin Phase 1.

Since cutting out all the foodstuffs I want you to avoid may be overwhelming, I am picking ONE thing for you to do each day, over the next 9 days. Talking about the slow and steady approach to your elimination diet will make it easier for you to adjust to *The Egg Quality Diet* eating plan.

KEY TIPS TO KEEP IN MIND DAILY

- Each day, be sure to drink about half your body weight in ounces of **filtered** water (but don't force yourself to drink if you're not thirsty)
- Each serving size of protein (fish or meat) is 3 ounces or about the size of your palm. Your goal is 70-80 grams of protein per day or approximately 10-12 ounces of protein daily (see the Protein Cheat Sheet in the resources section for tips on achieving this)
- Each serving size of vegetable is ½ cup of cooked vegetables. Your goal is 6-8 servings (or 3-4 cups) of cooked vegetables daily.
- Be sure to get in ½ ounce (or 15 grams) of grass fed liver in each day (or 3-4 ounces/90-120 grams per week). You can accomplish this by taking liver supplements (which can be found on AimeeRaupp.com/EQDiet) or eating liver pate (recipe on p. 332)
- It is important to keep your blood sugar balanced throughout your day, so do not go longer than 3-4 hours between eating meals/snacks
- If you have a known allergy to a certain food in the meal plan, please don't eat it
- If you get hungry, have ½ of a smoothie, grab an extra fat bomb or have some more carbohydrates in the form of sweet potato or plantain chips or grab one of the On The Go snacks listed in your reference sheet (making sure to pay attention to

which phase you're in and what's allowed in that phase)

- If you're in doubt of your macronutrients, use the MyFitnessPal app to track them daily until you get into a rhythm reminder your goal is approximately 45% fat, 30% protein, and 25% carbs (it's ok to be +/- a few percentage points on these macros)
- You'll notice we don't give exact measurements of food on the daily meal plans. Assume all serving sizes are 3-4 ounces (or the size of your palm) of proteins like meat and fish and that all vegetables are approximately 2-3 servings (1- 1 ½ cups of *cooked vegetables)* per meal or snack.
- Remember the meals we have laid out are a FRAMEWORK. If there is an ingredient you don't love, replace it with another similar and allowed ingredient within the phase of this plan you are in (i.e. you hate smoked salmon but love sardines, make the switch. Or you love beets but not asparagus, make the switch).
- Take time to meditate and/or journal each day about all the ways your body and your fertility are awakening. Head to AimeeRaupp.com/EQDiet for some of my guided meditations and mental/emotional exercises to get the most out of this plan.
- And, don't overlook the importance of sleep (it's ideal to get 7-8 hours nightly) and exercise (it's ideal to move your body 30-45 minutes 5-7 days/week).
- Have fun!

DAY ONE (Phase 1)

GOAL:

- Read all labels of the foods you eat and limit your ADDED sugar (remember, fruit sugars don't count) to under 10 grams/day.
- You will also avoid ALL artificial sweeteners.

Common Names for Added Sugar (your goal is to stay below 10 grams of added sugar):

Agave nectar	Brown sugar	Cane crystals
Cane sugar	Corn sweetener	Corn syrup
Crystalline fructose	Dextrose	Evaporated cane juice
Fructose	Glucose	Fruit juice concentrates
Lactose	Invert sugar	High-fructose corn syrup
Maltose	Malt syrup	Raw sugar
Sucrose	Syrup	

Common names for artificial sweeteners that you need to avoid:

Nutrasweet	Aspartame	Cyclamate
Canderel	AmnioSweet	Maltitol
Mannitol	Saccharin	Sorbitol
Xylitol	Sunette	Equal

Breakfast: two scrambled eggs with tomato, spinach, and fresh basil, a piece of bacon, and a slice of sweet potato toast

Snack: ½ cup of organic blueberries mixed with 1 tablespoon of Vital Proteins Collagen Peptides in 2 ounces of full-fat coconut milk (blend it and make a mini smoothie!)

Lunch: mixed mesclun green salad with wild salmon, avocado, green beans, olives, olive oil, and apple cider vinegar.

Snack: banana and two handfuls of almonds

Dinner: baked chicken with rosemary and lemon, sautéed kale with garlic, and half of a sweet potato with ghee.

DAY TWO (Phase 1)

GOAL:

- Continue limiting added sugar to less than 10mg a day
- Eliminate artificial sweeteners
- PLUS Eliminate soy

What avoiding soy looks like:

This means you are to avoid foodstuffs like soy cheese, soy milk, soy yogurt, soy sauce, tamari, and tofu. As well, look for these other sneaky soy ingredients and avoid them too:

Hydrolyzed soy protein
Hydrolyzed vegetable protein
Soy flour
Soy oil
Soy protein isolate
Textured vegetable protein (TVP)
Vegetable oil (this is usually soy oil)

Again, read labels and ditch ALL the foods in your home that contain soy, added sugars, and artificial sweeteners. I encourage you to throw these foods out (or donate them to a local shelter or church) because I never want you eating soy again. If you happen to have some fermented and non genetically modified soy products like miso, tempeh, or sprouted tofu AND you really enjoy eating them, find a safe place to hide these foods and you can try them again after week twelve of *The Egg Quality Diet*.

Breakfast: two hard-boiled eggs and a ½ cup of blueberries and a handful of almonds.

Snack: ½ cup of hummus with celery

Lunch: 2 organic, grass-fed, gluten-free sausages (chicken, pork, turkey) sautéed in coconut oil or ghee with coconut oil roasted beets

Snack: apple with almond butter

Dinner: beef tenderloin with sautéed bok choy, garlic, and spinach. Flavor with juice from half a lemon and a dash of sea salt.

DAY THREE (Phase 1)

GOAL:

- Continue limiting added sugar to less than 10mg a day
- Eliminate artificial sweeteners
- Eliminate soy
- PLUS Eliminate processed vegetable oils (because they are highly inflammatory)

Common names for processed vegetable oils are:

Canola oil

Cottonseed oil

Palm kernel oil (however Red Palm Oil is fine!)

Rapeseed oil

Shortening

Sunflower oil

Corn oil

Margarine

Peanut oil

Safflower oil

Soybean oil

What you will notice in eliminating processed and refined vegetable oils is that you will start avoiding almost all packaged foods. However, there are still some yummy packaged foods that are egg quality friendly and they're all listed in your On The Go Snack Idea hack sheet on page 59 (you can also find this hack sheet on AimeeRaupp.com/EQDiet).

Breakfast: coconut milk smoothie: 2-3 ounces of full-fat coconut milk, 1 tablespoon of almond butter, ½ avocado, ½ cup of strawberries, 1 tablespoon of Vital Proteins Collagen Peptides, and 2-3 ounces of water (depending on how you like your shakes).

Snack: ½ LARA bar

Lunch: mesclun green salad with grilled chicken, avocado, mushrooms (shitake, maitake, or black), olive oil, and vinegar. Flavor with some fresh ground pepper.

Snack: ½ cup of hummus with celery

Dinner: Pan sautéed filet of sole with shallots and leeks, roasted kale with rosemary and olive oil, and steamed asparagus. Garnish with the juice from a half of lemon.

DAY FOUR (Phase 1)

GOAL:

- Continue limiting added sugar to less than 10mg a day
- Eliminate artificial sweeteners
- Eliminate soy
- Eliminate processed vegetable oils
- PLUS Eliminate beans and legumes

Beans and legumes (as well as nuts and seeds) contain lectins, phytic acid and are a FODMAP food (meaning that they contain a type of carbohydrate called galacto-oligosaccharides that can cause unpleasant digestive problems for some people, especially people who already have IBS or similar digestive problems). Removing beans and legumes means you will remove all of the following from your diet (and put them in an out of sight place in your pantry):

Alfalfa
Beans (all varieties)
Carob
Chickpea
Clover
Field pea or garden pea
Lentil
Peanuts
Soybeans

As I discuss in my book Body Belief, legumes (aka beans) are highly inflammatory due to the lectins and phytic acid they contain. In order for you to allow your gut to heal, your immune system to regulate, and your fertility to truly thrive, you must avoid all beans from now until we reintroduce them (but, only when they're soaked & sprouted) in week nine of this eating plan.

Breakfast: two eggs over-easy with half an avocado

Snack: one grapefruit and one handful (about one ounce) of almonds

Lunch: grilled salmon with steamed broccoli and simple sauerkraut (make a full batch now, you'll use it throughout the program). Garnish with cracked pepper.

Snack: ½ cup of organic blueberries mixed with 1 tablespoon of flax seeds, 1 tablespoon of Vital Proteins Collagen Peptides in 2 ounces of full-fat coconut milk (blend it and make a mini smoothie!)

Dinner: quinoa pasta (or brown rice pasta—make sure the ingredients are just quinoa or brown rice no other flours) tossed in ghee and egg, topped with sautéed broccoli and grilled shrimp.

DAY FIVE (Phase 1)

GOAL:

- Continue limiting added sugar to less than 10mg a day
- Eliminate artificial sweeteners
- Eliminate soy
- Eliminate processed vegetable oils
- Eliminate beans and legumes
- PLUS Eliminate gluten and grains (yes, all grains as many people have an inflammatory reaction to grains of all types)

Yes, it's time to cut out gluten and grains. That means you are going to avoid ALL of the following gluten-containing grains AND all other grains and pseudograins (and remove them from your pantry as well *or hide them for now*):

Barley	Broths (boxed/store-bought)	Communion wafers
Einkorn	Farina	Graham
Kamut	Matzo	Processed meats Seitan
Soy sauce	Stock cubes	Triticale
Wheat germ	Bulgur	Couscous
Emmer	Farro	Imitation meats Marinades/sauces
MSG	Rye	Semolina

Spelt	Wheat	Textured vegetable protein(TVP)
Amaranth	Buckwheat	Chia seeds
Corn	Job's tears	Millet
Montina (Indian rice grass)	Oats	Quinoa
Rice (brown, white, and wild)	Teff	Sorghum

Going entirely grain-free can be tough at first. Yes, I will admit it...it can be tough but it can be majorly transformative to the health of your body. What helps me is eating carbohydrate-rich foods like plantains and sweet potatoes. Try some plantain chips or power balls from the recipe section at the back of this book (there are also some approved store-bought brands mentioned on the snacks hack sheet on page 59)

Breakfast: one fried egg with sauteed greens, one piece of bacon, and a grapefruit.

Snack: apple with almond butter

Lunch: mixed green salad with salmon, ½ of an avocado, tomato, olives, simple sauerkraut, olive oil, and vinegar.

Snack: ½ Larabar

Dinner: 2 organic, grass-fed sausages (chicken, pork, turkey) sauteed with organic tomato served with a side of steamed asparagus.

DAY SIX (Phase 1)

GOAL:

- Continue limiting added sugar to less than 10mg a day
- Eliminate artificial sweeteners
- Eliminate soy
- Eliminate processed vegetable oils
- Eliminate beans and legumes
- Eliminate gluten and grains
- PLUS Eliminate dairy (anything that contains lactose or casein can be inflammatory for many people)

As of today, you will be nixing the dairy- in every form:

Butter
Milk
Cheese
Yogurt
Ice cream

If you want to read more about how dairy, gluten, and grains impact inflammation and autoimmunity, head to AimeeRaupp.com/EQDiet and check out the resources I have for you on this topic.

Breakfast: Sunrise Hash

Snack: ½ Larabar

Lunch: grilled salmon and sauteed kale

Snack: coconut milk yogurt with blueberries

Dinner: Philly Steak Lettuce Cups and Baked Sweet Potato with ghee

DAY SEVEN (Phase 1)

GOAL:

- Continue limiting added sugar to less than 10mg a day
- Eliminate artificial sweeteners
- Eliminate soy
- Eliminate processed vegetable oils
- Eliminate beans and legumes
- Eliminate gluten and grains
- Eliminate dairy
- PLUS eliminate nightshades
- PLUS if you drink alcohol, today is your last day of drinking

You have probably heard this before: nightshade vegetables can be highly inflammatory. In fact, in my clinical practice, next to beans and legumes I see the biggest reduction in inflammation when my clients remove nightshades from their diet.

Nightshade vegetables are:

Ashwagandha

Bell peppers (sweet peppers)

Cayenne peppers

Curry mixes (the ones that contain any of these nightshade vegetables or seasonings) Eggplant

Goji berries

Hot peppers

Naranjillas

Paprika

> Pepinos
> Pimentos
> Tamarillos
> Tomatillos
> Tomatoes
> White potatoes (sweet potatoes are OK to eat)
>
> Skip all of these for now and try reintroducing them as directed in Phase 4.

Breakfast: Plantain Waffles and fresh berries

Snack: EPIC Bison Cranberry Bar

Lunch: Avocado Chicken Salad

Snack: baked sweet potato with simple sauerkraut

Dinner: baked salmon and sauteed broccoli

DAY EIGHT (Phase 1)

GOAL:

- Limiting added sugar to less than 10mg a day
- Eliminate artificial sweeteners
- Eliminate soy
- Eliminate processed vegetable oils
- Eliminate beans and legumes
- Eliminate gluten and grains
- Eliminate dairy
- Eliminate nightshades
- PLUS eliminate alcohol
- PLUS eliminate egg whites (because they contain lysozyme and protease inhibitors which can exacerbate intestinal permeability aka leaky gut)
- And, today is your last day of coffee. In the days that follow you can still have some caffeine, just no coffee. You will completely eliminate all caffeine for only a few days in Phase 2.

Breakfast: Plantain Pancakes topped with fresh berries

Snack: 6-8 oz. Kombucha and a medium sweet potato with cultured ghee

Lunch: Sweet Potato Toast topped with mashed avocado and over-easy egg

Snack: Key Lime Pie Fat Bombs

Dinner: Chicken Marbella and steamed swiss chard

DAY NINE (Phase 1)

GOAL:

- Limiting added sugar to less than 10mg a day
- Eliminate artificial sweeteners
- Eliminate soy
- Eliminate processed vegetable oils
- Eliminate beans and legumes
- Eliminate gluten and grains
- Eliminate dairy
- Eliminate nightshades
- Eliminate alcohol
- Eliminate egg whites
- PLUS eliminate coffee
- PLUS eliminate nuts and seeds (because like beans and legumes they contain phytic acid and lectins and can be highly inflammatory especially when consumed on a regular basis)
- PLUS breathe and cheer yourself on because you are a rockstar!

Breakfast: Coconut Porridge

Snack: Coconut Turmeric Bites

Lunch: Veggie Stir Fry with Shrimp

Snack: EPIC Bison Cranberry Bar

Dinner: Grilled Salmon and sauteed kale

CHAPTER FOUR

Phase 2
(11 days; partial week 2 & week 3)

Wow! You go! You have made it through the first Phase of *The Egg Quality Diet* and I am so proud of you! I hope you are feeling proud of yourself. Now, you will head into what is surely the most intense part of this diet, Phase 2. But, I know you can do it because I am giving you the step-by-step plan which will set you up for success. Phase 2 is all about purifying and detoxifying your body. The benefits for you: ultimate gut healing and renewing all the cells in your body including the ones in your uterus and ovaries (yes, all your cells!). This is where the real work starts. Key steps that are especially important for Phase 2 (these are in addition to your weekly tips as listed on page 64) are:

- This phase's mantra is: **Out with the old, in with the new.** Repeat this mantra to yourself often. Even better, write it out on a post-it and stick it where you will see it.
- Consume 6-8 ounces of liver support soup daily (recipe on page 282 and hack sheet on page 56). You will see this listed under a snack section during each day's meal plan but you can consume it whenever it works best for you (you will find the recipe, along with a few hacks in the recipe section of this book). *For some, when this soup is first introduced it can cause some detoxification symptoms (like a headache or loose bowels or feeling tired and sluggish; if that happens to you then cut back to 3-4 ounces and slowly increase to the recommended daily intake of 6-8 ounces)*

- When it comes to protein, refer to The Egg Quality Diet Guide, and in Phase 2 only consume wild salmon, wild cod, grass-fed beef, or lamb. Once you are in Phase 3 you can broaden your protein varieties.
- When it comes to vegetables, refer to The Egg Quality Diet Guide, and in Phase 2 only consume spinach, kale, broccoli, asparagus, cauliflower, sweet potatoes, butternut squash, sea vegetables, dandelion greens, or beets. NOTE: carrots are in the Liver Support Soup but only consume them in that recipe during Phase 2 as they are high in sugar.
- For seasoning, your food, refer to The Egg Quality Diet Guide, and in Phase 2 only consume parsley, ginger, turmeric, cinnamon, cilantro, or pink Himalayan sea salt.
- If you are taking vitamins and supplements, I typically recommend that you stop them for the duration of Phase 2 (which is 11 days). This is a great time to give your body a break from all the supplements *plus* it will give you time to reassess which supplements are best for your body and which supplements may actually be contributing to any kinks in your system (for a complete list of the supplements I have found best for fertility, head over to AimeeRaupp.com/ EQDiet). **IF YOU ARE ON ANY DOCTOR-PRESCRIBED MEDICATIONS, DO NOT STOP TAKING THEM.**
- Do a daily soak in the bath or a foot soak with a half cup of magnesium or Epsom salts
- Use magnesium oil on your body before bed. It comes in liquid form, use 8-10 sprays on any soft skin area of your body (i.e. abdomen or thighs) or your feet. Avoid your eyes. See which brands I like on AimeeRaupp.com/EQDiet
- Keep the daily tips mentioned below in mind
- Take a moment at the beginning of this week to honestly fill out your Kinks In Your Body Questionnaire (found on page

21 and also available for download at AimeeRaupp.com/ EQDiet)

- You will have FUN at the foodstore buying all of your favorite fertility healing foods (if you're like me and do your food shopping on Sundays, then print out this week's shopping list on page 217 and head to your grocery store!)
- You will continue to clean out your kitchen and pantry and get rid of all the foods that don't support your health or fertility
- You will continue to become reacquainted with your kitchen and begin cooking more
- You will continue to be easy on yourself and head to AimeeRaupp.com/EQDiet for more support if you need it
- Keep in mind, **Phase 2** of this plan, which is the strictest phase, the inflammation in your body will begin to dramatically shift. Due to that, you may not feel your best for the first few days of this Phase as you will be detoxing. For the best ways to support yourself in this Phase make sure you are staying hydrated with plenty of filtered water and add in a hot bath with 1-2 cups of Epsom or magnesium salts.
- Most of my clients feel amazing in this but Phase, but that's not always the case as everyone's body is so different. If you are one of the rare cases that are experiencing MORE digestive issues (like gas or bloating especially upper abdomen bloat) OR some of your red flag symptoms are getting worse, NOT better, please head to page 229 and read about histamines and SIBO and follow the tips laid out there to help you feel better.

Phase 2 Menu

REMEMBER: This is just a template for you to use, you can continue to eat your foods of choice as long as you eliminate the recommended foodstuffs as directed for each day.

All the recipes and shopping lists you need are in the back of this book (shopping lists are also on AimeeRaupp.com/EQDiet where you can download them and print them out for ease when doing your weekly food shopping).

KEY TIPS TO KEEP IN MIND DAILY

- Each day, be sure to drink about half your body weight in ounces of **filtered** water (but don't force yourself to drink if you aren't thirsty)
- Each serving size of protein (fish or meat) is 3 ounces or about the size of your palm. Your goal is 70-80 grams of protein per day or approximately 10-12 ounces of protein daily (see the Protein Cheat Sheet in the resources section for tips on achieving this)
- Each serving size of vegetable is ½ cup of cooked vegetables. Your goal is 6-8 servings (or 3-4 cups) of vegetables daily.
- Be sure to get in ½ ounce (or 15 grams) of grass fed liver in each day (or 3-4 ounces/90-120 grams per week). You can accomplish this by taking liver supplements (which can be found on AimeeRaupp.com/EQDiet) or eating liver pate (recipe on p. 332)

- It is important to keep your blood sugar balanced throughout your day, so do not go longer than 3-4 hours between eating meals/snacks
- If you have a known allergy to a certain food in the meal plan, please don't eat it
- If you get hungry, have ½ of a smoothie or grab an extra fat bomb or have some more carbohydrates in the form of sweet potato or plantain chips or grab one of the On The Go snacks listed in your reference sheet
- If you're in doubt of your macronutrients, use the MyFitnessPal app to track them daily until you get into a rhythm reminder your goal is approximately 45% fat, 30% protein, and 25% carbs
- You'll notice we don't give exact measurements of food on the daily meal plans. Assume all serving sizes are 3-4 ounces (or the size of your palm) of proteins like meat and fish and that all vegetables are approximately 2-3 servings (1- 1 ½ cups of *cooked vegetables)* per meal or snack
- Take time to meditate and/or journal each day about all the ways your body and your fertility are awakening. Head to AimeeRaupp.com/EQDiet for some of my guided meditations and mental/emotional exercises to get the most out of this plan.
- And, don't overlook the importance of sleep (it's ideal to get 7-8 hours nightly) and exercise (it's ideal to move your body 30-45 minutes 5-7 days/week).

DAY TEN (Phase 2)

If you have a craving during the day you may have one tablespoon serving of the Coconut Turmeric Bites or one of the Key Lime Pie or one of the Lemony fat bombs per day in Phase 2.

Upon waking, make yourself a mug of fresh ginger tea with the juice from half a lemon squeezed into it *or* a mug of hot water with a shot of apple cider vinegar or juice from half a lemon squeezed into it. You can also have some caffeine in the form of organic black or green or white tea; just keep it to one cup maximum.

Breakfast:
Coconut Milk Yogurt with Cinnamon

Snack:
6-8 oz. Kombucha and a sweet potato with cultured ghee
6-8 oz. Liver Support Soup

Lunch:
Grilled Wild Salmon and Asparagus sauteed with coconut oil, pink Himalayan sea salt, turmeric, and ginger. Add a squeeze of lemon to finish. (Make two servings to have one for dinner)

Snack:
Butternut Squash Soup with avocado

Dinner:
Grilled Wild Cod and Asparagus
4 oz. Bone Broth of your choice with one egg yolk

DAY ELEVEN (Phase 2)

If you have a craving during the day you may have one of the Coconut Turmeric Bites or one of the Key Lime Pie fat bombs per day in Phase 2.

Upon waking, make yourself a mug of fresh ginger tea with the juice from half a lemon squeezed into it *or* a mug of hot water with a shot of apple cider vinegar or juice from half a lemon squeezed into it. You can also have some caffeine in the form of organic black or green or white tea; just keep it to one cup maximum.

Breakfast:
Golden Milk Bone Broth

Snack:
Phase 2 Smoothie
Liver Support Soup

Lunch:
Grilled Steak with Spinach and Kale sauteed in cultured ghee with pink Himalayan sea salt (make two servings so you can have one for dinner)

Snack:
Yolk Ocado

Dinner:
Grilled Steak with Spinach and Kale
4 oz. Bone Broth of your choice

DAY TWELVE (Phase 2)

If you have a craving during the day you may have one of the Coconut Turmeric Bites or one of the Key Lime Pie fat bombs per day in Phase 2.

Upon waking, make yourself a mug of fresh ginger tea with the juice from half a lemon squeezed into it *or* a mug of hot water with a shot of apple cider vinegar or juice from half a lemon squeezed into it. You can also have some caffeine in the form of organic black or green or white tea; just keep it to one cup maximum.

Breakfast:
Phase 2 Smoothie

Snack:
Butternut Squash Soup

Lunch:
Grilled Cod with Broccoli and Cauliflower sauteed in coconut oil with turmeric (make two servings so you can have one for dinner)
Liver Support Soup

Snack:
½ c. Simple Sauerkraut and a sweet potato with cultured ghee

Dinner:
Grilled Cod with Broccoli and Cauliflower
4 oz. Bone Broth of your choice

DAY THIRTEEN (Phase 2)

If you have a craving during the day you may have one of the Coconut Turmeric Bites or one of the Key Lime Pie fat bombs per day in Phase 2.

Upon waking, make yourself a mug of fresh ginger tea with the juice from half a lemon squeezed into it *or* a mug of hot water with a shot of apple cider vinegar or juice from half a lemon squeezed into it. You can also have some caffeine in the form of organic black or green or white tea; just keep it to one cup maximum.

Breakfast:
Bone Broth Egg Drop Soup

Snack:
Phase 2 Smoothie
Liver Support Soup

Lunch:
Grilled Lamb and beets sauteed with coconut oil (make two servings for dinner)

Snack:
½ c. Simple Sauerkraut and sweet potato with cultured ghee

Dinner:
Grilled Lamb and beets
4 oz. Bone Broth of your choice

DAY FOURTEEN (Phase 2)

If you have a craving during the day you may have one of the Coconut Turmeric Bites or one of the Key Lime Pie fat bombs per day in Phase 2.

Upon waking, make yourself a mug of fresh ginger tea with the juice from half a lemon squeezed into it *or* a mug of hot water with a shot of apple cider vinegar or juice from half a lemon squeezed into it. You can also have some caffeine in the form of organic black or green or white tea; just keep it to one cup maximum.

Breakfast:
Coconut Milk Yogurt with Cinnamon

Snack:
Yolk Ocado and ½ c. of simple sauerkraut
Liver Support Soup

Lunch:
Butternut Squash Soup

Snack:
Ginger Turmeric Bone Broth

Snack:
Phase 2 Smoothie

Dinner:
Golden Milk Bone Broth
4 oz Bone Broth of your choice

DAY FIFTEEN (Phase 2)

KEEP IN MIND, THE NEXT FOUR DAYS YOU ARE EATING MAINLY BROTH/LIQUID FOODS. DO YOUR BEST TO FOLLOW THE MEAL PLAN EXACTLY AS LAID OUT FOR THE NEXT FOUR DAYS (which also means not all of the daily tips will be achieved, that is ok as you'll get back to meeting all the requirements in a few days). Over these four days, you are making a major impact on the health of your gut lining and setting the stage for ultimate healing and thriving.

Upon waking, make yourself a mug of fresh ginger tea with the juice from half a lemon squeezed into it *or* a mug of hot water with a shot of apple cider vinegar or juice from half a lemon squeezed into it. THERE IS NO CAFFEINE AT ALL TODAY.

Breakfast:
Golden Milk Bone Broth

Snack:
6-8 oz. Kombucha (please keep added sugars from kombucha to less than 5 grams/serving) and sweet potato with cultured ghee
Liver Support Soup

Lunch:
Bone Broth Egg Drop Soup

Snack:
Ginger Turmeric Bone Broth

Snack:

Phase 2 Smoothie

Dinner:

Butternut Squash Soup

4 oz. Bone Broth of your choice

DAY SIXTEEN (Phase 2)

Upon waking, make yourself a mug of fresh ginger tea with the juice from half a lemon squeezed into it *or* a mug of hot water with a shot of apple cider vinegar or juice from half a lemon squeezed into it. THERE IS NO CAFFEINE AT ALL TODAY.

Breakfast:
Phase 2 Smoothie

Snack:
½ cup simple sauerkraut and a sweet potato with cultured ghee
Liver Support Soup

Lunch:
Bone Broth Egg Drop Soup

Snack:
Ginger Turmeric Bone Broth

Snack:
Golden Milk Bone Broth

Dinner:
Butternut Squash Soup
4 oz. Bone Broth of your choice

DAY SEVENTEEN (Phase 2)

Upon waking, make yourself a mug of fresh ginger tea with the juice from half a lemon squeezed into it *or* a mug of hot water with a shot of apple cider vinegar or juice from half a lemon squeezed into it. THERE IS NO CAFFEINE AT ALL TODAY.

Breakfast:
Bone Broth Egg Drop Soup

Snack:
½ cup simple sauerkraut and a sweet potato with cultured ghee
Liver Support Soup

Lunch:
Butternut Squash Soup with ½ avocado

Snack:
Phase 2 Smoothie

Dinner:
Golden Milk Bone Broth
4 oz. Bone Broth of your choice

DAY EIGHTEEN (Phase 2)

Upon waking, make yourself a mug of fresh ginger tea with the juice from half a lemon squeezed into it *or* a mug of hot water with a shot of apple cider vinegar or juice from half a lemon squeezed into it. THERE IS NO CAFFEINE AT ALL TODAY.

Breakfast:
Coconut Milk Yogurt with Cinnamon

Snack:
Butternut Squash Soup
Liver Support Soup

Lunch:
Yolk Ocado and 4 ounces of bone broth of your choice

Snack:
½ cup simple sauerkraut and a sweet potato with cultured ghee

Dinner:
Phase 2 smoothie
4 oz. Bone Broth of your choice with one egg yolk

DAY NINETEEN (Phase 2)

Upon waking, make yourself a mug of fresh ginger tea with the juice from half a lemon squeezed into it *or* a mug of hot water with a shot of apple cider vinegar or juice from half a lemon squeezed into it. You can add in some caffeine today and future days but it must be either organic black, green, or white tea.

Breakfast:
Golden Milk Bone Broth

Snack:
Phase 2 Smoothie
Liver Support Soup

Lunch:
Grilled Steak with Spinach and Kale sauteed in cultured ghee with pink Himalayan sea salt (make two servings so you can have one for dinner)

Snack:
Yolk Ocado and simple sauerkraut

Dinner:
Grilled Steak with Spinach and Kale
4 oz. Bone Broth of your choice

DAY TWENTY (Phase 2)

Upon waking, make yourself a mug of fresh ginger tea with the juice from half a lemon squeezed into it *or* a mug of hot water with a shot of apple cider vinegar or juice from half a lemon squeezed into it.

Breakfast:
Phase 2 Smoothie

Snack:
Butternut Squash Soup

Lunch:
Grilled Cod with Broccoli and Cauliflower sauteed in coconut oil with turmeric (make two servings so you can have one for dinner)
Liver Support Soup

Snack:
½ c. Simple Sauerkraut and a sweet potato with cultured ghee

Dinner:
Grilled Cod with Broccoli and Cauliflower
4 oz. Bone Broth of your choice with one egg yolk

CHAPTER FIVE

Phase 3 (weeks 4- 7)

BOOM! You just made it through Phase 2, which I think is the most challenging phase of this diet. Give yourself a massive hug as you have just made a tremendous impact on the state of inflammation in your body, your gut health, and your egg quality! We are now headed into four weeks of Phase 3. In Phase 1 and 2 you laid the groundwork for a healthier gut, immune system, and hormones and Phase 3 is going to make that work stick. As you move through the four weeks of Phase 3, your cells are turning over and being replaced by stronger ones with thriving mitochondrial function, the lining of your gut is becoming less inflamed and more receptive to all the good nutrients you are feeding it and your immune system is loving your body and all it's inner workings more and more. The kinks in your system are receding and you are creating a dream environment for your baby to come into. And, queue the dance party because you can now reintroduce:

- Your supplements and vitamins (if you want to know the fertility supplements I recommend the most, head to AimeeRaupp.com/EQDiet)
- Fruit
  - You can have 6-8 servings per week of low sugared fruit: melons, berries, and grapefruit
  - You can have 2-4 servings per week of moderate to high sugared fruits: apples, apricots, kiwi, nectarine, papaya, plum, pomegranate, pears, peach, citrus (all of them except grapefruit, which is low sugared), banana, mango, pineapple, plantains, watermelon, dates, and fresh figs

- o When it comes to dried fruit and fruit juices, they are very high in sugar and I don't typically recommend them unless consumed sparingly (meaning once every two weeks or less)
- You can broaden your protein sources to any grass-fed/pastured meat and any wild-caught or Seafood Watch approved seafood (keeping a special eye on how you react to shellfish). Head to the resources section in this book and/or AimeeRaupp.com/EQDiet to see the latest information on the best seafood in your area. Also, keep in mind:
  - o I recommend 6-10 servings per week of meat
  - o I recommend 8-12 servings per week of fish
- You can broaden your vegetable sources, adding in all vegetables EXCEPT for nightshade vegetables (as listed on page 79). Also as I mentioned at the beginning of Phase 2: Most of my clients feel amazing by this point in the protocol, but that's not always the case as everyone's body is so different. If you are one of the rare cases that are experiencing MORE digestive issues (like gas or bloating especially upper abdomen bloat) OR some of your red flag symptoms are getting worse, NOT better, please head to page 229 and read about histamines and SIBO and follow the tips laid out there to help you feel better.
- You can have 1 cup of caffeine daily in the form of organic black, green or white tea
- You will remain in Phase 3 for four weeks as this amount of time is crucial to healing your gut, balancing hormones, and regulating your immune system. At the end of the four weeks, you will begin to reintroduce, in a systematic fashion, many of the foods that you eliminated back in Phase 1.
- Keep it up with your regular servings of liver support soup. Ideally, you are having 4-6 ounces 5-7 times/week.

- Keep the daily tips listed below in mind as you move through the next month
- Don't forget to fill out your Kinks questionnaire (you can download it on AimeeRaupp.com/EQDiet) on a weekly basis so you can best monitor how your body is shifting and healing.
- Also, we have a new mantra for week one of Phase 3: I am renewing, every single cell in my body is renewing. Repeat this mantra to yourself often. Even better, write it out on a post-it and stick it where you will see it. With each new week of this Phase 3, I will be giving you a new mantra and some weekly tips on how to best succeed on this plan. Here's where I am going to begin to layer in some other important tools for maximizing fertility.

Phase 3 (Week 4) Menu

REMEMBER: This is just a template for you to use, you can continue to eat your foods of choice as long as you eliminate the recommended foodstuffs as directed for each day.

All the recipes and shopping lists you need are in the back of this book (shopping lists are also on AimeeRaupp.com/EQDiet where you can download them and print them out for ease when doing your weekly food shopping).

KEY TIPS TO KEEP IN MIND DAILY

- Each day, be sure to drink about half your body weight in ounces of **filtered** water (but don't force yourself to drink if you're not thirsty)
- Each serving size of protein (fish or meat) is 3 ounces or about the size of your palm. Your goal is 70-80 grams of protein per day or approximately 10-12 ounces of protein daily (see the Protein Cheat Sheet in the resources section for tips on achieving this)
- Each serving size of vegetable is ½ cup of cooked vegetables. Your goal is 6-8 servings (or 3-4 cups) of vegetables daily.
- Be sure to get in ½ ounce (or 15 grams) of grass fed liver in each day (or 3-4 ounces/90-120 grams per week). You can accomplish this by taking liver supplements (which can be found on

AimeeRaupp.com/EQDiet) or eating liver pate (recipe on p. 332)

- It is important to keep your blood sugar balanced throughout your day, so do not go longer than 3-4 hours between eating meals/snacks
- If you have a known allergy to a certain food in the meal plan, please don't eat it
- If you get hungry, have ½ of a smoothie or grab an extra fat bomb or have some more carbohydrates in the form of sweet potato or plantain chips or grab one of the On The Go snacks listed on page 59
- If you're in doubt of your macronutrients, use the MyFitnessPal app to track them daily until you get into a rhythm reminder your goal is approximately 45% fat, 30% protein, and 25% carbs
- You'll notice we don't give exact measurements of food on the daily meal plans. Assume all serving sizes are 3-4 ounces (or the size of your palm) of proteins like meat and fish and that all vegetables are approximately 2-3 servings (1- 1 ½ cups of *cooked vegetables)* per meal or snack
- Take time to meditate and/or journal each day about all the ways your body and your fertility are awakening. Head to AimeeRaupp.com/EQDiet for some of my guided meditations and mental/ emotional exercises to get the most out of this plan.
- And, don't overlook the importance of sleep (it's ideal to get 7-8 hours nightly) and exercise (it's ideal to move your body 30-45 minutes 5-7 days/week).

Weekly Tip For Success:

Going forward we want to make sure that you are set up for success. Anyone who has made any dietary or lifestyle change will tell you that your best chance to succeed is by planning and being prepared. There's nothing worse than being hungry and realizing you have nothing safe to eat in the house! This week we are going to batch cook. That means that some of these recipes (I'll mark them with an asterisk) are going to make a bigger batch than we've done so far. Don't be intimidated- you've already been batch cooking your bone broth and some of the soups we've made from bone broth and you didn't even know it. You're going to freeze the extra servings and you'll reheat as needed in the oven. Freezing stops the histamine production so freeze anything you won't be using in the next two days.

Your Mantra For This Week:

I am renewing, every single cell in my body is renewing.

DAY TWENTY-ONE (Phase 3; week 4)

Upon waking, make yourself a mug of fresh ginger tea with the juice from half a lemon squeezed into it *or* a mug of hot water with a shot of apple cider vinegar or juice from half a lemon squeezed into it. Now that you have entered Phase 3 you may also have one cup of organic black or green tea or white tea today.

Breakfast:
Morning Smoothie

Snack:
Bone Broth Egg Drop Soup
Liver Support Soup

Lunch:
Sweet Potato Toast with Mashed Avocado and 4 oz. bone broth of your choice

Snack:
Golden Milk Bone Broth and a ½ cup simple sauerkraut

Dinner:
Grilled Cod with Zoodles and NoMato Sauce
4 oz. bone broth of your choice

DAY TWENTY-TWO (Phase 3; week 4)

Upon waking, make yourself a mug of fresh ginger tea with the juice from half a lemon squeezed into it *or* a mug of hot water with a shot of apple cider vinegar or juice from half a lemon squeezed into it. You may also have one mug of organic black or green tea today.

Breakfast:
Ham and White Sweet Potato Hash* (would be delicious with hollandaise sauce)

Snack:
Butternut Squash Soup
Liver Support Soup

Lunch:
Deconstructed Egg Rolls*

Snack:
Ginger Turmeric Bone Broth and simple sauerkraut

Dinner:
Grilled Salmon and sauteed asparagus with hollandaise sauce
4 oz. Bone Broth of your choice with one egg yolk

DAY TWENTY-THREE (Phase 3; week 4)

Upon waking, make yourself a mug of fresh ginger tea with the juice from half a lemon squeezed into it *or* a mug of hot water with a shot of apple cider vinegar or juice from half a lemon squeezed into it. You may also have one mug of organic black or green tea today.

Breakfast:
Breakfast Casserole

Snack:
Golden Milk Bone Broth and simple sauerkraut
Liver Support Soup

Lunch:
Thai Coconut Soup*

Snack:
Yolk Ocado

Dinner:
Grilled Steak with Broccoli and Cauliflower sauteed in coconut oil
4 oz. Bone Broth of your choice

DAY TWENTY-FOUR (Phase 3; week 4)

Upon waking, make yourself a mug of fresh ginger tea with the juice from half a lemon squeezed into it *or* a mug of hot water with a shot of apple cider vinegar or juice from half a lemon squeezed into it. You may also have one mug of organic black or green tea today.

Breakfast:
Coconut Milk Yogurt with cinnamon

Snack:
Red Beet and Apple Salad

Lunch:
Sweet Potato Toast with mashed avocado and grilled fish of choice
Liver Support Soup

Snack:
Bone Broth Egg Drop Soup

Dinner:
Shrimp Scampi
4 oz. Bone Broth of your choice

DAY TWENTY-FIVE (Phase 3; week 4)

Upon waking, make yourself a mug of fresh ginger tea with the juice from half a lemon squeezed into it *or* a mug of hot water with a shot of apple cider vinegar or juice from half a lemon squeezed into it. You may also have one mug of organic black or green tea today.

Breakfast:
Morning Smoothie

Snack:
Ginger Turmeric Bone Broth

Lunch:
Pork and Bok Choy Stir Fry* with Coconut Cauliflower Rice*
Liver Support Soup

Snack:
½ c. simple sauerkraut and a sweet potato with cultured ghee

Dinner:
Grilled Cod with sauteed asparagus and leeks and hollandaise sauce
4 oz. Bone Broth of your choice with one egg yolk

DAY TWENTY-SIX (Phase 3; week 4)

Upon waking, make yourself a mug of fresh ginger tea with the juice from half a lemon squeezed into it *or* a mug of hot water with a shot of apple cider vinegar or juice from half a lemon squeezed into it. You may also have one mug of organic black or green tea today.

Breakfast:
Mango Mint Green Smoothie

Snack:
Bone Broth Egg Drop Soup
Liver Support Soup

Lunch:
Sweet Potato Toast with Mashed Avocado and grilled fish of choice

Snack:
Golden Milk Bone Broth

Dinner:
One-Dish Roasted Brats with Apples and Butternut Squash*
4 oz. bone broth of your choice

DAY TWENTY-SEVEN (Phase 3; week 4)

Upon waking, make yourself a mug of fresh ginger tea with the juice from half a lemon squeezed into it *or* a mug of hot water with a shot of apple cider vinegar or juice from half a lemon squeezed into it. You may also have one mug of organic black or green tea today.

Breakfast:
Coconut Milk Yogurt with cinnamon

Snack:
Butternut Squash Soup

Lunch:
Grilled Salmon and sauteed asparagus with hollandaise sauce
Liver Support Soup

Snack:
Ginger Turmeric Bone Broth

Dinner:
Coconut Baked Shrimp with Arugula, Avocado and Grapefruit Salad
4 oz. Bone Broth of your choice

DAY TWENTY-EIGHT (Phase 3; week 4)

Upon waking, make yourself a mug of fresh ginger tea with the juice from half a lemon squeezed into it *or* a mug of hot water with a shot of apple cider vinegar or juice from half a lemon squeezed into it. You may also have one mug of organic black or green tea today.

Breakfast:
Sunrise Hash and berries of choice

Snack:
Golden Milk Bone Broth
Liver Support Soup

Lunch:
Butternut Squash Soup and grilled fish of choice

Snack:
Yolk Ocado and simple sauerkraut

Dinner:
Grilled fish of choice with Broccoli and Cauliflower sauteed in coconut oil
4 oz. Bone Broth of your choice

Phase 3 (Week 5 Menu)

Weekly Tip For Success:

You are one week into Phase 3, and you are rocking it! You are now laying the groundwork for sustainable gut healing and hormone balancing so stay the course. For this week, don't forget to do your weekly tips (as listed on page 104). You'll also notice that we no longer have a detailed weekly shopping list, now we have a shopping list template for you (found on page 225 and also on AimeeRaupp.com/EQDiet). I want you to feel empowered to create your own meal plans if you want to venture from the plan as set. Your core shopping list will always include bone broth ingredients, plenty of green leafy vegetables and root veggies, and your chosen grass-fed, wild-caught, or pastured proteins. Then you'll add the ingredients you need based on your pantry stock and the recipes you're choosing to cook each week.

Last week we focused more on batch cooking and for the rest of Phase 3 (weeks five, six & seven) we're going to ramp that up. Sometimes it will be making extras of a whole recipe and other times we'll just make an extra protein that will serve in another recipe later in the week. You're going to freeze the extra servings and you'll reheat as needed in the oven. Freezing stops the histamine production so freeze anything you won't be using in the next two days. And, consume any leftovers in the refrigerator within two days to keep the histamine load down (need to know more about histamines? Head to the resources section and read up on how histamines can impact fertility).

Your Mantra For This Week:

I am whole. I am fertile.

DAY TWENTY-NINE (Phase 3; week 5)

Upon waking, make yourself a mug of fresh ginger tea with the juice from half a lemon squeezed into it *or* a mug of hot water with a shot of apple cider vinegar or juice from half a lemon squeezed into it. You may also have one mug of organic black or green tea today.

Breakfast:
Coconut Milk Yogurt with cinnamon

Snack:
Red Beet and Apple Salad

Lunch:
Sweet Potato Toast with mashed avocado and 4 oz. bone broth
Liver Support Soup

Snack:
Bone Broth Egg Drop Soup and simple sauerkraut

Dinner:
Shrimp Scampi with zoodles
4 oz. Bone Broth of your choice

DAY THIRTY (Phase 3; week 5)

Upon waking, make yourself a mug of fresh ginger tea with the juice from half a lemon squeezed into it *or* a mug of hot water with a shot of apple cider vinegar or juice from half a lemon squeezed into it. You may also have one mug of organic black or green tea today.

Breakfast:
Sunrise Hash

Snack:
Ginger Turmeric Bone Broth

Lunch:
Grilled Cod with sauteed asparagus and leeks and hollandaise sauce
Liver Support Soup

Snack:
½ c. simple sauerkraut and a sweet potato with cultured ghee

Dinner:
Beef Stroganoff* over Baked Sweet Potatoes
4 oz. Bone Broth of your choice

DAY THIRTY-ONE (Phase 3; week 5)

Upon waking, make yourself a mug of fresh ginger tea with the juice from half a lemon squeezed into it *or* a mug of hot water with a shot of apple cider vinegar or juice from half a lemon squeezed into it. You may also have one mug of organic black or green tea today.

Breakfast:
Choose your favorite smoothie recipe

Snack:
Butternut Squash Soup and simple sauerkraut
Liver Support Soup

Lunch:
Vietnamese Spring Rolls and Broccoli Salad with Cranberries

Snack:
Ginger Turmeric Bone Broth

Dinner:
Beef Barbacoa Bowls (reserve extra beef for tomorrow night, no need to freeze)
4 oz. Bone Broth of your choice

DAY THIRTY-TWO (Phase 3; week 5)

Upon waking, make yourself a mug of fresh ginger tea with the juice from half a lemon squeezed into it *or* a mug of hot water with a shot of apple cider vinegar or juice from half a lemon squeezed into it. You may also have one mug of organic black or green tea today.

Breakfast:
Maple Chicken Breakfast Sausage and Avocado

Snack:
Golden Milk Bone Broth

Lunch:
Stir-Fried Greens with Sausage and Roasted Beets

Snack:
Yolk Ocado

Dinner:
Shredded Beef Tacos with Mango Salsa and Roasted Root Veggies (use extra beef from the previous night)
4 oz. Bone Broth of your choice

DAY THIRTY-THREE (Phase 3; week 5)

Upon waking, make yourself a mug of fresh ginger tea with the juice from half a lemon squeezed into it *or* a mug of hot water with a shot of apple cider vinegar or juice from half a lemon squeezed into it. You may also have one mug of organic black or green tea today.

Breakfast:
Fruit Salad and Bacon (throw together your favorite fruit and your favorite bacon, easy peasy)

Snack:
Bone Broth Egg Drop Soup and simple sauerkraut
Liver Support Soup

Lunch:
Sweet Potato Toast with mashed avocado and grilled fish of choice

Snack:
Matcha Latte and coconut yogurt

Dinner:
Slow Cooker Ham (takes six hours on low- plan ahead) and leftover Roasted Root Veggies
4 oz. Bone Broth of your choice

DAY THIRTY-FOUR (Phase 3; week 5)

Upon waking, make yourself a mug of fresh ginger tea with the juice from half a lemon squeezed into it *or* a mug of hot water with a shot of apple cider vinegar or juice from half a lemon squeezed into it. You may also have one mug of organic black or green tea today.

Breakfast:
Ham and Eggs (warm some leftover ham from last night and prepare eggs however you'd like)

Snack:
Yolk Ocado
Liver Support Soup

Lunch:
Grilled fish of choice with sauteed kale

Snack:
½ c. simple sauerkraut and a sweet potato with cultured ghee

Dinner:
Grilled Cod with sauteed asparagus and leeks and hollandaise sauce
4 oz. Bone Broth of your choice

DAY THIRTY-FIVE (Phase 3; week 5)

Upon waking, make yourself a mug of fresh ginger tea with the juice from half a lemon squeezed into it *or* a mug of hot water with a shot of apple cider vinegar or juice from half a lemon squeezed into it. You may also have one mug of organic black or green tea today.

Breakfast:
Garden Green Brothie

Snack:
Bone Broth Egg Drop Soup
Liver Support Soup

Lunch:
Sweet Potato Toast with Mashed Avocado and grilled fish of choice

Snack:
Golden Milk Bone Broth

Dinner:
Vietnamese Spring Rolls and Broccoli Salad with Cranberries (leftover from earlier in the week)
4 oz. bone broth of your choice

Phase 3 (week 6) Menu

Weekly Tip For Success:

OK, I am hoping you feel like you have this Phase 3 thing down pat. And that you are noticing many changes to the symptoms of inflammation you had at the beginning of this 100-day program (remember, you're supposed to be filling out that Kinks questionnaire on a weekly basis to keep yourself in the loop on yourself and your symptoms). This week will be more of the same when it comes to batch cooking and freezing your food. As you have likely learned, preparation is the key to success with this diet. So keep at it as we have two more weeks to go in Phase 3, and then we get to start adding back in some of the foods you have missed. Don't forget to do your weekly tips (as listed on page 104) and use your shopping list template if you need to. For this week. I also want you to put aside time to watch my video on the 5 Simple Ways To Improve Your Fertility Naturally. One of the tips is diet, which you have covered in this book, but the other tips are really important for you to learn about as well. This video is also on the AimeeRaupp.com/EQDiet but here is the link as well: https://www.youtube.com/watch?v=GFzrYd8fb98

Your Mantra For This Week:

My body and all of its cells are reawakening.

DAY THIRTY-SIX (Phase 3; week 6)

Upon waking, make yourself a mug of fresh ginger tea with the juice from half a lemon squeezed into it *or* a mug of hot water with a shot of apple cider vinegar or juice from half a lemon squeezed into it. You may also have one mug of organic black or green tea today.

Breakfast:
Maple Chicken Sausage with Fruit Salad

Snack:
Butternut Squash Soup with simple sauerkraut
Liver Support Soup

Lunch:
Grilled fish of choice with veggies

Snack:
Ginger Turmeric Bone Broth

Dinner:
Shredded Beef Tacos with Mango Salsa and Roasted Root Veggies
4 oz. Bone Broth of your choice with one egg yolk

DAY THIRTY-SEVEN (Phase 3; week 6)

Upon waking, make yourself a mug of fresh ginger tea with the juice from half a lemon squeezed into it *or* a mug of hot water with a shot of apple cider vinegar or juice from half a lemon squeezed into it. You may also have one mug of organic black or green tea today.

Breakfast:
Choose your favorite smoothie recipe

Snack:
Butternut Squash Soup
Liver Support Soup

Lunch:
Turkey and Bacon Rollups with Radish Salad

Snack:
Ginger Turmeric Bone Broth with simple sauerkraut

Dinner:
40 Clove Chicken and spinach sauteed in ghee (no need to freeze extra chicken, you're using it tomorrow)
4 oz. Bone Broth of your choice with one egg yolk

DAY THIRTY-EIGHT (Phase 3; week 6)

Upon waking, make yourself a mug of fresh ginger tea with the juice from half a lemon squeezed into it *or* a mug of hot water with a shot of apple cider vinegar or juice from half a lemon squeezed into it. You may also have one mug of organic black or green tea today.

Breakfast:
Breakfast Hash and eggs

Snack:
Golden Milk Bone Broth and simple sauerkraut
Liver Support Soup

Lunch:
Spaghetti Zoodles with Faux-Mato Bolognese

Snack:
Yolk Ocado

Dinner:
Chicken and Asparagus Stir Fry (use chicken from yesterday)
4 oz. Bone Broth of your choice

DAY THIRTY-NINE (Phase 3; week 6)

Upon waking, make yourself a mug of fresh ginger tea with the juice from half a lemon squeezed into it *or* a mug of hot water with a shot of apple cider vinegar or juice from half a lemon squeezed into it. You may also have one mug of organic black or green tea today.

Breakfast:
Fruit Bowl with Coconut Butter and side of Bacon

Snack:
Bone Broth Egg Drop Soup and simple sauerkraut
Liver Support Soup

Lunch:
Sweet Potato Toast with mashed avocado and grilled fish of choice

Snack:
Matcha Latte and coconut yogurt

Dinner:
Tuna Over Kale and Roasted Root Veggies
4 oz. Bone Broth of your choice

DAY FORTY (Phase 3; week 6)

Upon waking, make yourself a mug of fresh ginger tea with the juice from half a lemon squeezed into it *or* a mug of hot water with a shot of apple cider vinegar or juice from half a lemon squeezed into it. You may also have one mug of organic black or green tea today.

Breakfast:
Coconut Milk Yogurt with Cinnamon and Berries

Snack:
Yolk Ocado
Liver Support Soup

Lunch:
Thai Coconut Soup with grilled fish of choice

Snack:
½ c. simple sauerkraut and a sweet potato with cultured ghee

Dinner:
Grilled Cod with sauteed asparagus and leeks and hollandaise sauce
4 oz. Bone Broth of your choice

DAY FORTY-ONE (Phase 3; week 6)

Upon waking, make yourself a mug of fresh ginger tea with the juice from half a lemon squeezed into it *or* a mug of hot water with a shot of apple cider vinegar or juice from half a lemon squeezed into it. You may also have one mug of organic black or green tea today.

Breakfast:
Morning Smoothie

Snack:
Bone Broth Egg Drop Soup
Liver Support Soup

Lunch:
Sweet Potato Toast with Mashed Avocado and grilled fish of choice

Snack:
Golden Milk Bone Broth and simple sauerkraut

Dinner:
Thai Crispy Pork Salad
4 oz. bone broth of your choice

Phase 3 (week 7) Menu

Your Weekly Tip For Success:

You are freaking rocking this! Week 7! Holy Moly! One more week to go, and we get to start reintroducing foods! This week, after doing your weekly Kinks questionnaire, I'd love for you to make a list of the 10-20 foods you miss the most. But be specific, i.e., instead of listing nuts, list the kind of nut (almonds, walnuts, etc.). Your list will be your guide to your very own reintroduction. You are about to create the best diet for you, your hormones, and those gorgeous eggs in your ovaries. After making your list, the rest of this week will be like the past few weeks… batch cooking and preparing yourself for success. Don't forget to do your weekly tips (for ease, I've listed them below) and use your shopping list template if you need to. REMEMBER: You are almost halfway through this program, and I hope you feel as amazing as you deserve. As an added weekly tip for this week, I invite you to learn more about doing castor oil packs and why they can help improve ovarian and uterine blood flow and help increase fertility. Watch this short video and learn more: https://youtu.be/e8JvoAlAr9o (this video can also be found on AimeeRaupp.com/EQDiet)

Your Mantra For This Week:

I am a rockstar, and I am proud of my body.

KEY TIPS TO KEEP IN MIND DAILY

- Each day, be sure to drink about half your body weight in ounces of **filtered** water (keeping in mind not to force yourself to drink if you are not thirsty)
- Each serving size of protein (fish or meat) is 3 ounces or about the size of your palm. Your goal is 70-80 grams of protein per day or approximately 10-12 ounces of protein daily (see the Protein Cheat Sheet in the resources section for tips on achieving this)
- Each serving size of vegetable is ½ cup of cooked vegetables. Your goal is 6-8 servings (or 3-4 cups) of vegetables daily.
- Be sure to get in ½ ounce (or 15 grams) of grass fed liver in each day (or 3-4 ounces/90-120 grams per week). You can accomplish this by taking liver supplements (which can be found on AimeeRaupp.com/EQDiet) or eating liver pate (recipe on p. 332)
- It is important to keep your blood sugar balanced throughout your day, so do not go longer than 3-4 hours between eating meals/snacks.
- If you have a known allergy to a certain food in the meal plan, please don't eat it
- If you get hungry, have ½ of a smoothie or grab an extra fat bomb or have some more carbohydrates in the form of sweet potato or plantain chips or grab one of the On The Go snacks listed in your reference sheet

- If you're in doubt of your macronutrients, use the MyFitnessPal app to track them daily until you get into a rhythm reminder your goal is approximately 45% fat, 30% protein, and 25% carbs
- You'll notice we don't give exact measurements of food on the daily meal plans. Assume all serving sizes are 3-4 ounces (or the size of your palm) of proteins like meat and fish and that all vegetables are approximately 2-3 servings (1- 1 ½ cups of *cooked vegetables*) per meal or snack
- Take time to meditate and/or journal each day about all the ways your body and your fertility are awakening. Head to AimeeRaupp.com/EQDiet for some of my guided meditations and mental/ emotional exercises to get the most out of this plan.
- And, don't overlook the importance of sleep (it's ideal to get 7-8 hours nightly) and exercise (it's ideal to move your body 30-45 minutes 5-7 days/week).

DAY FORTY-TWO (Phase 3; week 7)

Upon waking, make yourself a mug of fresh ginger tea with the juice from half a lemon squeezed into it *or* a mug of hot water with a shot of apple cider vinegar or juice from half a lemon squeezed into it. You may also have one mug of organic black or green tea today.

Breakfast:
Beth's Berry Brothie

Snack:
Butternut Squash Soup with simple sauerkraut
Liver Support Soup

Lunch:
Grilled fish of choice with veggies

Snack:
Ginger Turmeric Bone Broth

Dinner:
Tuna Over Kale and a Sweet Potato (or leftover roasted veggies)
4 oz. Bone Broth of your choice

DAY FORTY-THREE (Phase 3; week 7)

Upon waking, make yourself a mug of fresh ginger tea with the juice from half a lemon squeezed into it *or* a mug of hot water with a shot of apple cider vinegar or juice from half a lemon squeezed into it. You may also have one mug of organic black or green tea today.

Breakfast:
Breakfast Hash and eggs

Snack:
Golden Milk Bone Broth with simple sauerkraut
Liver Support Soup

Lunch:
40 Clove Chicken and Sauteed Spinach (leftovers)

Snack:
Yolk Ocado

Dinner:
Spaghetti Zoodles with Faux-Mato Bolognese (leftovers)
4 oz. Bone Broth of your choice

DAY FORTY-FOUR (Phase 3; week 7)

Upon waking, make yourself a mug of fresh ginger tea with the juice from half a lemon squeezed into it *or* a mug of hot water with a shot of apple cider vinegar or juice from half a lemon squeezed into it. You may also have one mug of organic black or green tea today.

Breakfast:
Sunrise Hash and eggs

Snack:
Butternut Squash Soup and simple sauerkraut
Liver Support Soup

Lunch:
Thai Crispy Pork Salad (leftover from late last week)

Snack:
Ginger Turmeric Bone Broth

Dinner:
Grilled fish of choice with veggies
4 oz. Bone Broth of your choice

DAY FORTY-FIVE (Phase 3; week 7)

Upon waking, make yourself a mug of fresh ginger tea with the juice from half a lemon squeezed into it *or* a mug of hot water with a shot of apple cider vinegar or juice from half a lemon squeezed into it. You may also have one mug of organic black or green tea today.

Breakfast:
Fruit Salad and a side of bacon

Snack:
Golden Milk Bone Broth and simple sauerkraut
Liver Support Soup

Lunch:
Zucchini Spinach Salad with Chicken

Snack:
Yolk Ocado

Dinner:
White Fish Packets with Zucchini and Summer Herbs
4 oz. Bone Broth of your choice

DAY FORTY-SIX (Phase 3; week 7)

Upon waking, make yourself a mug of fresh ginger tea with the juice from half a lemon squeezed into it *or* a mug of hot water with a shot of apple cider vinegar or juice from half a lemon squeezed into it. You may also have one mug of organic black or green tea today.

Breakfast:
Coconut Yogurt with cinnamon and fruit

Snack:
Bone Broth Egg Drop Soup and simple sauerkraut
Liver Support Soup

Lunch:
Sweet Potato Toast with mashed avocado and grilled fish of choice

Snack:
Matcha Latte and coconut yogurt

Dinner:
Grilled Sole with Asparagus and Broccoli sauteed in ghee
4 oz. Bone Broth of your choice

DAY FORTY-SEVEN (Phase 3; week 7)

Upon waking, make yourself a mug of fresh ginger tea with the juice from half a lemon squeezed into it *or* a mug of hot water with a shot of apple cider vinegar or juice from half a lemon squeezed into it. You may also have one mug of organic black or green tea today.

Breakfast:
Sunrise Hash and kombucha

Snack:
Yolk Ocado
Liver Support Soup

Lunch:
Grilled fish of choice with sauteed spinach and kale

Snack:
½ c. simple sauerkraut and a sweet potato with cultured ghee

Dinner:
Zucchini Spinach Salad with Chicken
4 oz. Bone Broth of your choice

DAY FORTY-EIGHT (Phase 3; week 7)

Upon waking, make yourself a mug of fresh ginger tea with the juice from half a lemon squeezed into it *or* a mug of hot water with a shot of apple cider vinegar or juice from half a lemon squeezed into it. You may also have one mug of organic black or green tea today.

Breakfast:
Mango Mint Smoothie

Snack:
Bone Broth Egg Drop Soup
Liver Support Soup

Lunch:
Sweet Potato Toast with Mashed Avocado and grilled fish of choice

Snack:
Golden Milk Bone Broth and simple sauerkraut

Dinner:
Whitefish Packets with Zucchini (leftovers)
4 oz. bone broth of your choice

DAY FORTY-NINE (Phase 3; week 7)

Upon waking, make yourself a mug of fresh ginger tea with the juice from half a lemon squeezed into it *or* a mug of hot water with a shot of apple cider vinegar or juice from half a lemon squeezed into it. You may also have one mug of organic black or green tea today.

Breakfast:
Phase 2 Smoothie

Snack:
Butternut Squash Soup and simple sauerkraut
Liver Support Soup

Lunch:
Turkey and Bacon Rollups with Radish Salad

Snack:
Ginger Turmeric Bone Broth

Dinner:
Ginger Lime Salmon Bowls
4 oz. Bone Broth of your choice and one egg yolk

Chapter Six

Phase 4 (weeks 8-15)

You made it to the last phase (Phase 4) of this plan and you are now officially halfway through *The Egg Quality Diet.* You are 50 days into your 100 day eating plan for better hormones, a happy gut, a balanced immune system, and a less inflamed body. You should be feeling proud of yourself and hopefully full of energy with glowing skin and brimming with fertility. At this point, I would expect (based on my clinical experience with this program) that 70-90% of the kinks you had on your first round of doing the Kinks In Your System Questionnaire should be gone. If that's not the case and you are not feeling as good as you think you should be, and you know you followed this diet as best as you could, please head to page 229 and read about histamines and SIBO (if neither of those issues seems like it fits you, you may consider staying in Phase 3 for a bit longer until more of your symptoms abate). If you are feeling great, then it is time to REINTRODUCE SOME FOODS! Get out that list you made at the beginning of last week (week 7) where you noted the top 10-20 foods you miss the most and let's start adding them in while *clearly following my instructions* on reintroducing foods.

How To Reintroduce Foods

You have worked hard the past 50 days and I want you, your hormones, your eggs, and your fertility to continue to benefit from all that you have done so please follow my guidance on how to properly reintroduce foods. A key step in the reintroduction phase is you staying connected to you and feeling all the feels. Sometimes a food reaction gives you a rash, sometimes it's bloating or gas, other times it's anxiety or a racing heart or insomnia. Use the food diary template we have for you on AimeeRaupp.com/EQDiet to really track what you ate and how you felt after eating it. As well, keep an eye on any of your previously noted kinks from your questionnaire and if they start to reappear then it's a signal from your body that what you have now reintroduced doesn't jive with the cells in your body and is causing unwanted inflammation. Because I can't be there with you as you reintroduce foods, you need to be your own detective here and pay close attention to any and all shifts in your system when you reintroduce foods.

OK, let's get out that list and pick your first item to reintroduce. I am going to break down for you exactly how to reintroduce foods in the sentences that follow but I also have it broken down in another way on the next page, as everyone learns differently and I want to make sure you reintroduce foods the right way so you can get the most out of this plan. My recommendation is to choose the food or food group you desire and have ½ a serving of that food two times on the first day, if you have any reactions (see the below list for common ones), don't have the food again. If you have no reactions then on the second day have a full serving of the food. If you have a reaction, don't have the food again. If you have no reactions on this second day and continue to have no reactions on the 3rd and 4th day after (don't eat the food again on the 3rd and 4th day, just monitor for symptoms) you are good to continue eating this food. When choosing which foods to reintroduce first, it is Ideal that you start with the least processed foods first-- things like sprouted nuts or seeds or sprouted beans or nightshade vegetables. After you've done some of those reintroductions successfully then you can move to foods like grains (ideally they're sprouted and organic) and then flours (ideally gluten-free and organic ones). Alcohol and caffeine can also be added back in as desired, but the key is to not reintroduce more than one new thing at a time AND don't reintroduce more than two new things in any 7 day period as it can take a few days for symptoms to show up. Symptoms to watch for include:

- Rashes and skin changes (like little pink bumps on your body)
- Hives
- Joint pain
- Headaches or migraines
- Increased mucus or phlegm
- Runny nose
- Sneezing
- Coughing and/or need to clear throat
- Fatigue
- Brain fog
- Dizziness
- Difficulty sleeping
- Changes in breathing
- Bloating
- Stomach pain or cramps
- Changes in bowel habits
- Racing heart or palpitations
- Anxiety
- Acne
- A return of any of your symptoms from the Kinks questionnaire

If you experience no symptoms during the period where you reintroduce a food group, you can assume that it is fine to eat and move on to the next food group. However, if you experience negative symptoms like those mentioned above, then you have successfully identified a trigger food and should remove it from your diet. Keep in mind, your body may just need some more healing time before it can tolerate certain foods. So if a food caused a trigger, I recommend keeping it out of your diet for the next 4-8 weeks and then trying it again to see if it still causes a trigger **(please keep in mind this advice does not pertain to foods you have a known allergy to as there is a very big difference between food intolerance and an anaphylactic reaction to a food. Consult with your doctor if you are unsure about this difference).**

Here's an example of what reintroduction of food looks like on a hypothetical week (you don't have to do this on a Monday, I'm just using that as an example starting day for ease):

Monday: reintroduce ½ serving of food in the morning and afternoon. Look for any symptoms. If you have a reaction, don't try this food again for 4-8 weeks.

Tuesday: If you don't have any reactions, have a full serving of the food in the morning and afternoon. Look for any symptoms. If you have a reaction, don't try this food again for 4-8 weeks.

Wednesday & Thursday: don't reintroduce anything new AND don't have any servings of the food you reintroduced on Monday and Tuesday. If there are no symptoms then this food is fine for you to add back to your diet. Now choose the next food to reintroduce the following day (Friday) and follow the same plan as outlined above. If there are symptoms, then mark them down in your journal along with the food that caused them and consider eliminating that food for good or revisiting the reintroduction of it in 4-8 weeks. If you move at the pace I've listed out for you then you should be able to have many of your favorite foods back in the mix in a month or two.

From my personal experience after doing this diet for the first time I learned that almonds (even when organic and sprouted or in nut butter or milk form) can flare up my eczema if I have them more than 3 times a week. So, I can still have almonds (in all forms) as long as I don't have them daily (like I used to). I notice that corn (even organic) causes me to have sleep disturbances, white potatoes give me gas, gluten and dairy constipate me and soy causes my whole body to revolt. I also found that my body does better on fewer grains overall and that the liver support soup is a key to keeping my body weight in check. All interesting findings for me as I've always been so in touch with my body. I'd also like to add that now that I know all of these different inflammatory reactions, I can pick and choose foods that work best for me and my body. And sometimes I can also choose to have the foods that I know give me a reaction, but at least I know what to expect when I do. Over time the conscious connection to the food reaction brings you to a place of choosing that food less often because feeling good feels so damn good.

Here are some important words on reintroducing foods from the author of *The Paleo Approach*, Sarah Ballantyne that I want you to take in fully:

"It's best not to be in a hurry to reintroduce foods. Generally, the longer you wait, the more likely you are to be successful. Ultimately, when you introduce particular foods is your choice. How you feel is the best gauge, and only you will know if you are ready. A word of caution, though: don't let cravings influence you. Your decision should be based on how good you feel and how much improvement you're seeing in your disease. Don't reintroduce a new food if you have an infection, have just had an unusually strenuous workout, got less sleep than normal, are feeling unusually stressed, or are under any other circumstances that may make interpreting a reaction

difficult. If you have a hard time determining which food causes what reaction, wait longer between reintroductions. Even if reintroduction is successful, you may wish to keep your consumption of the food to a minimum (like reserving a glass of wine for Sunday dinner) for the best long-term results. The foods you tolerate may change over time, so a failed reintroduction does not mean you can never eat that food again. Some foods that you reintroduce will also be relegated to "sometimes foods." These will include alcohol and potentially some of the stage 4 reintroductions, like gluten-free grains. Sometimes food is one that doesn't cause a reaction when you consume it occasionally, but that can subtly undermine your health (even if simply by displacing more nutrient-dense options) if you consume it on a regular basis. These are still worth reintroducing, even if they aren't going to make it into your normal rotation because they give you more flexibility in situations like travel and eating out."[16]

For the full article on this topic, check out the resources section of this book

Living in Phase 4

As you move into Phase 4 of this plan, your body is still healing and renewing and the inflammation is subsiding so continue to follow the plan as best you can. The goal is to remain in Phase 4 for the next 50 days (just about 8 weeks) so that you achieve optimum results and top-quality eggs. When living in this phase and reintroducing foods come at it with a sense of curiosity, asking yourself: How does this food best support my body and my goals? How do I feel when I eat this food? Tuning into not only physical reactions to food but also emotional ones. Ultimately, *The Egg Quality Diet* is about teaching you how to nourish yourself. I think you will get the most out of this book and its plan when you approach from the space of you taking care of you (P.S. so many of the offerings on AimeeRaupp.com/EQDiet will really help you nourish and care for yourself on every level- mentally, emotionally, physically and nutritionally; so make sure you're taking advantage of all those resources).

As you will see, the menu I have laid out for Phase 4 is your template (along with your shopping lists at the back of the book and on AimeeRaupp.com/EQDiet). It is up to you to add to the template laid out herein any of the foods you have reintroduced. With each new week in Phase 4, I will continue to give you weekly encouragement and mantras as well I will continue to highlight an important lifestyle tip or educational tool to help you to continue to maximize your fertility and egg quality.

Weekly Tip For Success:
Follow the reintroduction steps I mapped out for you. Have fun and be curious. Continue to batch cook and try new recipes from

this book. Listen to your body and tune in to how it's feeling and how it's reacting to any new foods you have brought into your diet. In addition, take some time this week to watch my video on the best exercise for you and your fertility: https://youtu.be/G-1MNjvC7tw (remember this video and so many other pieces of educational material are available to you on AimeeRaupp.com/EQDiet)

Your Mantra For The Week: I love & support my body and my body loves & supports me back. We are a team.

KEY TIPS TO KEEP IN MIND DAILY

- Each day, be sure to drink about half your body weight in ounces of **filtered** water (keeping in mind not to force yourself to drink if you are not thirsty)
- Each serving size of protein (fish or meat) is 3 ounces or about the size of your palm. Your goal is 70-80 grams of protein per day or approximately 10-12 ounces of protein daily (see the Protein Cheat Sheet in the resources section for tips on achieving this)
- Each serving size of vegetable is ½ cup of cooked vegetables. Your goal is 6-8 servings (or 3-4 cups) of vegetables daily.
- Be sure to get in ½ ounce (or 15 grams) of grass fed liver in each day (or 3-4 ounces/90-120 grams per week). You can accomplish this by taking liver supplements (which can be found on AimeeRaupp.com/EQDiet) or eating liver pate (recipe on page 332)

148

- It is important to keep your blood sugar balanced throughout your day, so do not go longer than 3-4 hours between eating meals/snacks
- If you have a known allergy to a certain food in the meal plan, please don't eat it
- If you get hungry, have ½ of a smoothie or grab an extra fat bomb or have some more carbohydrates in the form of sweet potato or plantain chips or grab one of the On The Go snacks listed in your reference sheet
- If you're in doubt of your macronutrients, use the MyFitnessPal app to track them daily until you get into a rhythm reminder your goal is approximately 45% fat, 30% protein, and 25% carbs
- You'll notice we don't give exact measurements of food on the daily meal plans. Assume all serving sizes are 3-4 ounces (or the size of your palm) of proteins like meat and fish and that all vegetables are approximately 2-3 servings (1- 1 ½ cups of *cooked vegetables)* per meal or snack
- Keep it up with your regular servings of liver support soup. Ideally, you are having 4-6 ounces 5-7 times/week.
- Take time to meditate and/or journal each day about all the ways your body and your fertility are awakening. Head to AimeeRaupp.com/EQDiet for some of my guided meditations and mental/ emotional exercises to get the most out of this plan.
- And, don't overlook the importance of sleep (it's ideal to get 7-8 hours nightly) and exercise (it's ideal to move your body 30-45 minutes 5-7 days/week).

Phase 4 (week 8) Menu

DAY FIFTY (Phase 4; week 8)

Upon waking, make yourself a mug of fresh ginger tea with the juice from half a lemon squeezed into it *or* a mug of hot water with a shot of apple cider vinegar or juice from half a lemon squeezed into it. You may also have one mug of organic black or green tea today.

Breakfast:
Eggs and fruit salad

Snack:
Golden Milk Bone Broth and simple sauerkraut
Liver Support Soup

Lunch:
Butternut Squash Soup and grilled fish

Snack:
Yolk Ocado

Dinner:
Grilled fish and roasted veggies
4 oz. Bone Broth of your choice

DAY FIFTY-ONE (Phase 4; week 8)

Upon waking, make yourself a mug of fresh ginger tea with the juice from half a lemon squeezed into it *or* a mug of hot water with a shot of apple cider vinegar or juice from half a lemon squeezed into it. You may also have one mug of organic black or green tea today.

Breakfast:
Maple Chicken Breakfast Sausage with Avocado

Snack:
Butternut Squash Soup and simple sauerkraut
Liver Support Soup

Lunch:
Mixed Veggie Noodles with Pork

Snack:
Ginger Turmeric Bone Broth

Dinner:
Pancit
4 oz. Bone Broth of your choice with one egg yolk

DAY FIFTY-TWO (Phase 4; week 8)

Upon waking, make yourself a mug of fresh ginger tea with the juice from half a lemon squeezed into it *or* a mug of hot water with a shot of apple cider vinegar or juice from half a lemon squeezed into it. You may also have one mug of organic black or green tea today.

Breakfast:
Breakfast Hash and eggs

Snack:
Golden Milk Bone Broth
Liver Support Soup

Lunch:
Avocado Chicken Salad

Snack:
Yolk Ocado and simple sauerkraut

Dinner:
Grilled Sole with Asparagus and Hollandaise
4 oz. Bone Broth of your choice

DAY FIFTY-THREE (Phase 4; week 8)

Upon waking, make yourself a mug of fresh ginger tea with the juice from half a lemon squeezed into it *or* a mug of hot water with a shot of apple cider vinegar or juice from half a lemon squeezed into it. You may also have one mug of organic black or green tea today.

Breakfast:

Sausage Patties, sauteed spinach, and mixed berries

Snack:

Bone Broth Egg Drop Soup and simple sauerkraut
Liver Support Soup

Lunch:

Sweet Potato Toast with Mashed Avocado and grilled fish

Snack:

Matcha Latte and coconut yogurt

Dinner:

Grilled fish of choice with roasted veggies
4 oz. Bone Broth of your choice

DAY FIFTY-FOUR (Phase 4; week 8)

Upon waking, make yourself a mug of fresh ginger tea with the juice from half a lemon squeezed into it *or* a mug of hot water with a shot of apple cider vinegar or juice from half a lemon squeezed into it. You may also have one mug of organic black or green tea today.

Breakfast:
Maple Chicken Breakfast Sausage with Avocado and mixed berries

Snack:
Yolk Ocado
Liver Support Soup

Lunch:
Vietnamese Spring Rolls and sauteed greens

Snack:
½ c. simple sauerkraut and a sweet potato with cultured ghee

Dinner:
Chinese Shredded Beef with Broccoli
4 oz. Bone Broth of your choice

DAY FIFTY-FIVE (Phase 4; week 8)

Upon waking, make yourself a mug of fresh ginger tea with the juice from half a lemon squeezed into it *or* a mug of hot water with a shot of apple cider vinegar or juice from half a lemon squeezed into it. You may also have one mug of organic black or green tea today.

Breakfast:

Breakfast Hash and eggs with mixed berries

Snack:

Bone Broth Egg Drop Soup and simple sauerkraut
Liver Support Soup

Lunch:

Grilled fish of choice with roasted veggies

Snack:

Golden Milk Bone Broth

Dinner:

Chicken, Broccoli, and Sweet Potato Sheet Pan Dinner
4 oz. bone broth of your choice

DAY FIFTY-SIX (Phase 4; week 8)

Upon waking, make yourself a mug of fresh ginger tea with the juice from half a lemon squeezed into it *or* a mug of hot water with a shot of apple cider vinegar or juice from half a lemon squeezed into it. You may also have one mug of organic black or green tea today.

Breakfast:
Morning Smoothie

Snack:
Butternut Squash Soup and simple sauerkraut
Liver Support Soup

Lunch:
Chinese Shredded Beef with Broccoli

Snack:
Ginger Turmeric Bone Broth

Dinner:
Grilled fish of choice with sauteed greens
4 oz. Bone Broth of your choice

Phase 4 (week 9) Menu & Weekly Tips

I hope your first week of reintroductions went well and you are feeling a little more adventurous in your diet. I also hope you are feeling more in touch with your body and how it responds to the food and nourishment you give it. Know that your gut is still healing, your eggs are still getting healthier and your hormones are becoming more and more balanced as each phase of this plan passes. Be proud of yourself!

Weekly Tip For Success:

Continue to follow the reintroduction steps as I mapped out for you (on page 141). Continue to have fun and be curious. Continue to batch cook and try new recipes from this book. Listen to your body and tune into how it's feeling and how it's reacting to any new foods you have brought into your diet. Make sure to continue to focus on the daily tips as listed on page 148. And get excited... by the end of this week, you could feasibly have 4 of your favorite foods back in your diet! For even more inspiration, head over to AimeeRaupp.com/EQDiet and watch my 3- part video series on how to naturally improve FSH and AMH, the crucial supplements for fertility, and how to release shame around your fertility challenges. You will love these videos for me as they are filled with so much incredible content.

Your Mantra For The Week: I am creating a beautiful vessel for my child to live in.

DAY FIFTY-SEVEN (Phase 4; week 9)

Upon waking, make yourself a mug of fresh ginger tea with the juice from half a lemon squeezed into it *or* a mug of hot water with a shot of apple cider vinegar or juice from half a lemon squeezed into it. You may also have one mug of organic black or green tea today.

Breakfast:
Sausage Patties with sauteed spinach and eggs

Snack:
Golden Milk Bone Broth and simple sauerkraut
Liver Support Soup

Lunch:
Butternut Squash Soup and grilled fish

Snack:
Yolk Ocado

Dinner:
Pancit
4 oz. Bone Broth of your choice

DAY FIFTY-EIGHT (Phase 4; week 9)

Upon waking, make yourself a mug of fresh ginger tea with the juice from half a lemon squeezed into it *or* a mug of hot water with a shot of apple cider vinegar or juice from half a lemon squeezed into it. You may also have one mug of organic black or green tea today.

Breakfast:

Mangu

Snack:

Bone Broth Egg Drop Soup and simple sauerkraut
Liver Support Soup

Lunch:

40 Clove Chicken and Cauliflower Rice

Snack:

Beth's Berry Brothie

Dinner:

Ginger Lime Salmon Bowls
4 oz. Bone Broth of your choice

DAY FIFTY-NINE (Phase 4; week 9)

Upon waking, make yourself a mug of fresh ginger tea with the juice from half a lemon squeezed into it *or* a mug of hot water with a shot of apple cider vinegar or juice from half a lemon squeezed into it. You may also have one mug of organic black or green tea today.

Breakfast:
Sausage and Butternut Squash Breakfast Skillet

Snack:
Red Beet and Apple Salad
Liver Support Soup

Lunch:
Chicken Soup with Roasted Veggies (use leftover chicken from yesterday's lunch)

Snack:
Golden Milk Bone Broth and simple sauerkraut

Dinner:
Grilled fish of choice and sauteed spinach or kale
4 oz. Bone Broth of your choice

DAY SIXTY (Phase 4; week 9)

Upon waking, make yourself a mug of fresh ginger tea with the juice from half a lemon squeezed into it *or* a mug of hot water with a shot of apple cider vinegar or juice from half a lemon squeezed into it. You may also have one mug of organic black or green tea today.

Breakfast:
Sweet Potato Blueberry Bacon Skillet

Snack:
Yolk Ocado and simple sauerkraut
Liver Support Soup

Lunch:
Grilled fish and veggies

Snack:
Coconut Milk Yogurt with berries

Dinner:
Sheet Pan Greek Chicken and veggies
4 oz. Bone Broth of your choice

DAY SIXTY-ONE (Phase 4; week 9)

Upon waking, make yourself a mug of fresh ginger tea with the juice from half a lemon squeezed into it *or* a mug of hot water with a shot of apple cider vinegar or juice from half a lemon squeezed into it. You may also have one mug of organic black or green tea today.

Breakfast:
Coconut Porridge

Snack:
Morning Smoothie
Liver Support Soup

Lunch:
Deconstructed Egg Rolls and Leftover Cauliflower Rice from earlier in the week

Snack:
Butternut Squash Soup and simple sauerkraut

Dinner:
Vietnamese Spring Rolls
4 oz. Bone Broth of your choice

DAY SIXTY-TWO (Phase 4; week 9)

Upon waking, make yourself a mug of fresh ginger tea with the juice from half a lemon squeezed into it *or* a mug of hot water with a shot of apple cider vinegar or juice from half a lemon squeezed into it. You may also have one mug of organic black or green tea today.

Breakfast:
Sunrise Hash and mixed berries

Snack:
Phase 2 Smoothie
Liver Support Soup

Lunch:
Grilled fish, sauteed greens, and simple sauerkraut

Snack:
Sweet Potato Toast and a scrambled egg

Dinner:
Grilled fish and roasted veggies
4 oz. Bone Broth of your choice

DAY SIXTY-THREE (Phase 4; week 9)

Upon waking, make yourself a mug of fresh ginger tea with the juice from half a lemon squeezed into it *or* a mug of hot water with a shot of apple cider vinegar or juice from half a lemon squeezed into it. You may also have one mug of organic black or green tea today.

Breakfast:
Plantain Waffles and sausage patties

Snack:
Epic bar
Liver Support Soup

Lunch:
Shepherd's Pie

Snack:
Yolk Ocado

Dinner:
Leftovers of your choice
4 oz. Bone Broth of your choice

Phase 4 (week 10) Menu & Weekly Tips

OK, now that you have the reintroduction routine down, over the next 6 weeks I am going to layer on some more fertility bonuses to help you achieve the success you are longing for a healthy fertile body that will bring home a healthy thriving baby. As I mentioned at the very beginning of this book- diet is just one piece of the puzzle when it comes to balanced hormones, optimal egg quality, and brimming fertility. The other components: mental/emotional, physical, and spiritual health also all play a significant role in your ability to get and to stay pregnant. Remember, I've been helping women bring home babies for almost 20 years and I know for certain that a woman can have the diet part down pat and still not get the results she wants. I am sure by now you have visited the website that goes with this book (AimeeRaupp.com/EQDiet) to download your shopping lists or see what supplements I recommend for fertility and maybe you've taken a look at some of the other offerings on that site. Each week for the next 6 weeks, in your weekly tips for success, I am going to highlight one of those non-diet-related offerings on AimeeRaupp.com/EQDiet so that you don't miss out on all the other fertility enhancing tools I have to offer you. This way, you can get all you need from me and my expertise. Also as we head into this week, make sure you are hitting all of your daily tips (as found on page 148).

Weekly Tip For Success:
As I mentioned above, moving forward these weekly tips for success are going to highlight some additional materials that I have created regarding how to best optimize health and fertility. This

week, I want to focus on understanding your genetics and how you can live your life in a way to amplify wellness over illness. Additionally, there is a very specific genetic mutation, called the MTHFR mutation, that affects many women who are trying to conceive. I am highlighting two videos where I teach you all about genetics and aging and how to best optimize your system, on all levels, for fertility. Head to AimeeRaupp.com/EQDiet and in the video library section and check out these two videos:

Epigenetics & Egg Quality: An Interview with Dr. Merhi
(reproductive endocrinologist): https://youtu.be/vf9guNnt5g4

Supplements for Fertility: MTHFR & Folic Acid:
https://youtu.be/zKo1NO3Uz80

Your Mantra For The Week: I am at ease in my life.

DAY SIXTY-FOUR (Phase 4; week 10)

Upon waking, make yourself a mug of fresh ginger tea with the juice from half a lemon squeezed into it *or* a mug of hot water with a shot of apple cider vinegar or juice from half a lemon squeezed into it. You may also have one mug of organic black or green tea today.

Breakfast:
Coconut Milk Yogurt with cinnamon and mixed berries

Snack:
Red Beet and Apple Salad

Lunch:
Sweet Potato Toast with mashed avocado and grilled fish of choice
Liver Support Soup

Snack:
Bone Broth Egg Drop Soup and simple sauerkraut

Dinner:
Shrimp Scampi with zoodles
4 oz. Bone Broth of your choice

DAY SIXTY-FIVE (Phase 4; week 10)

Upon waking, make yourself a mug of fresh ginger tea with the juice from half a lemon squeezed into it *or* a mug of hot water with a shot of apple cider vinegar or juice from half a lemon squeezed into it. You may also have one mug of organic black or green tea today.

Breakfast:
Sunrise Hash and eggs

Snack:
Ginger Turmeric Bone Broth

Lunch:
Grilled Cod with sauteed asparagus and leeks and hollandaise sauce
Liver Support Soup

Snack:
½ c. simple sauerkraut and a sweet potato with cultured ghee

Dinner:
Veggie Stir Fry with Shrimp
4 oz. Bone Broth of your choice

DAY SIXTY-SIX (Phase 4; week 10)

Upon waking, make yourself a mug of fresh ginger tea with the juice from half a lemon squeezed into it *or* a mug of hot water with a shot of apple cider vinegar or juice from half a lemon squeezed into it. You may also have one mug of organic black or green tea today.

Breakfast:

Plantain Waffles (freeze leftovers for next week) and side of berries

Snack:

Butternut Squash Soup and simple sauerkraut
Liver Support Soup

Lunch:

Vietnamese Spring Rolls and Broccoli Salad with Cranberries

Snack:

Ginger Turmeric Bone Broth

Dinner:

Beef Barbacoa Bowls (reserve extra beef for tomorrow night, no need to freeze)
4 oz. Bone Broth of your choice

DAY SIXTY-SEVEN (Phase 4; week 10)

Upon waking, make yourself a mug of fresh ginger tea with the juice from half a lemon squeezed into it *or* a mug of hot water with a shot of apple cider vinegar or juice from half a lemon squeezed into it. You may also have one mug of organic black or green tea today.

Breakfast:
Maple Chicken Breakfast Sausage and Avocado

Snack:
Golden Milk Bone Broth and simple sauerkraut
Liver Support Soup

Lunch:
Stir-Fried Greens with Sausage and Roasted Beets

Snack:
Yolk Ocado

Dinner:
Shredded Beef Tacos with Mango Salsa and Roasted Root Veggies (use extra beef from the previous night)
4 oz. Bone Broth of your choice

DAY SIXTY-EIGHT (Phase 4; week 10)

Upon waking, make yourself a mug of fresh ginger tea with the juice from half a lemon squeezed into it *or* a mug of hot water with a shot of apple cider vinegar or juice from half a lemon squeezed into it. You may also have one mug of organic black or green tea today.

Breakfast:

Fruit Salad and Bacon (throw together your favorite fruit and your favorite bacon, easy peasy)

Snack:

Bone Broth Egg Drop Soup and simple sauerkraut
Liver Support Soup

Lunch:

Sweet Potato Toast with mashed avocado and grilled fish of choice

Snack:

Matcha Latte and coconut yogurt

Dinner:

Slow Cooker Ham (takes six hours on low- plan ahead) and leftover Roasted Root Veggies
4 oz. Bone Broth of your choice

DAY SIXTY-NINE (Phase 4; week 10)

Upon waking, make yourself a mug of fresh ginger tea with the juice from half a lemon squeezed into it *or* a mug of hot water with a shot of apple cider vinegar or juice from half a lemon squeezed into it. You may also have one mug of organic black or green tea today.

Breakfast:

Ham and Eggs (warm some leftover ham from last night and prepare eggs however you'd like)

Snack:

Yolk Ocado

Liver Support Soup

Lunch:

Sweet potato and grilled fish of choice

Snack:

½ c. simple sauerkraut and a sweet potato with cultured ghee

Dinner:

Grilled Cod with sauteed asparagus and leeks and hollandaise sauce

4 oz. Bone Broth of your choice

DAY SEVENTY (Phase 4; week 10)

Upon waking, make yourself a mug of fresh ginger tea with the juice from half a lemon squeezed into it *or* a mug of hot water with a shot of apple cider vinegar or juice from half a lemon squeezed into it. You may also have one mug of organic black or green tea today.

Breakfast:
Garden Green Brothie

Snack:
Bone Broth Egg Drop Soup
Liver Support Soup

Lunch:
Sweet Potato Toast with Mashed Avocado and 4 oz. bone broth of your choice

Snack:
Golden Milk Bone Broth

Dinner:
Vietnamese Spring Rolls and Broccoli Salad with Cranberries (leftover from earlier in the week)
4 oz. bone broth of your choice

Phase 4 (week 11) Menu & Weekly Tips

You are cruising through *The Egg Quality Diet* and I'm trusting that you're feeling great. At this point, I'd suspect most of the kinks in your system have been worked out. Also, be sure to keep an eye that you aren't seeing some of your symptoms (aka kinks) creep back in as you add in more foods. If you feel like there's been a setback, take a week off from reintroducing foods so you can assess what is going on in your body. However, if you're still feeling good, then keep trying out foods and see how you feel. P.S. Don't forget to keep following all of the daily tips as listed on page 148.

Weekly Tip For Success:
This week I want to highlight the importance of healthy sperm. Not every one of you reading this book is in a heterosexual relationship. So if sperm health isn't something you need to worry about because you are using a donor and you know the sperm is good quality, you can skip this week's tip for success. But, if you are in a heterosexual partnership and want to know more ways to improve sperm health, check out these tools I have for you (reminder, all of these tools are also linked out on AimeeRaupp.com/EQDiet):

Improving Sperm Quality with the Healthy Daddy Diet: **https://youtu.be/uqdTAi2gBhQ**

5 Tips To Optimize Sperm Health:
https://www.youtube.com/watch?v=tj-yvv5giGY&t=2s

Your Mantra For The Week: Everything I need is on its way to me.

DAY SEVENTY-ONE (Phase 4; week 11)

Upon waking, make yourself a mug of fresh ginger tea with the juice from half a lemon squeezed into it *or* a mug of hot water with a shot of apple cider vinegar or juice from half a lemon squeezed into it. You may also have one mug of organic black or green tea today.

Breakfast:
Maple Chicken Sausage and eggs with Fruit Salad

Snack:
Butternut Squash Soup
Liver Support Soup

Lunch:
Grilled Fish with sauteed greens and simple sauerkraut

Snack:
Ginger Turmeric Bone Broth

Dinner:
Shredded Beef Tacos with Mango Salsa and Roasted Root Veggies
4 oz. Bone Broth of your choice

DAY SEVENTY-TWO (Phase 4; week 11)

Upon waking, make yourself a mug of fresh ginger tea with the juice from half a lemon squeezed into it *or* a mug of hot water with a shot of apple cider vinegar or juice from half a lemon squeezed into it. You may also have one mug of organic black or green tea today.

Breakfast:
Plantain Waffles and fruit salad

Snack:
Butternut Squash Soup
Liver Support Soup

Lunch:
Turkey and Bacon Roll-Ups with Radish Salad

Snack:
Ginger Turmeric Bone Broth and simple sauerkraut

Dinner:
40 Clove Chicken and spinach sauteed in ghee (no need to freeze extra chicken, you're using it tomorrow)
4 oz. Bone Broth of your choice

DAY SEVENTY-THREE (Phase 4; week 11)

Upon waking, make yourself a mug of fresh ginger tea with the juice from half a lemon squeezed into it *or* a mug of hot water with a shot of apple cider vinegar or juice from half a lemon squeezed into it. You may also have one mug of organic black or green tea today.

Breakfast:
Breakfast Hash

Snack:
Golden Milk Bone Broth
Liver Support Soup

Lunch:
Veggie Stir Fry with Shrimp

Snack:
Yolk Ocado and simple sauerkraut

Dinner:
Chicken and Asparagus Stir Fry (use chicken from yesterday)
4 oz. Bone Broth of your choice

DAY SEVENTY-FOUR (Phase 4; week 11)

Upon waking, make yourself a mug of fresh ginger tea with the juice from half a lemon squeezed into it *or* a mug of hot water with a shot of apple cider vinegar or juice from half a lemon squeezed into it. You may also have one mug of organic black or green tea today.

Breakfast:
Fruit Bowl with Coconut Butter and side of Bacon

Snack:
Bone Broth Egg Drop Soup and simple sauerkraut
Liver Support Soup

Lunch:
Sweet Potato Toast with mashed avocado and grilled fish

Snack:
Matcha Latte and coconut yogurt

Dinner:
Tuna Over Kale and Roasted Root Veggies
4 oz. Bone Broth of your choice

DAY SEVENTY-FIVE (Phase 4; week 11)

Upon waking, make yourself a mug of fresh ginger tea with the juice from half a lemon squeezed into it *or* a mug of hot water with a shot of apple cider vinegar or juice from half a lemon squeezed into it. You may also have one mug of organic black or green tea today.

Breakfast:
Coconut Milk Yogurt with Cinnamon and Berries

Snack:
Yolk Ocado
Liver Support Soup

Lunch:
Grilled fish and roasted veggies

Snack:
½ c. simple sauerkraut and a sweet potato with cultured ghee

Dinner:
Grilled Cod with sauteed asparagus and leeks and hollandaise sauce
4 oz. Bone Broth of your choice

DAY SEVENTY-SIX (Phase 4; week 11)

Upon waking, make yourself a mug of fresh ginger tea with the juice from half a lemon squeezed into it *or* a mug of hot water with a shot of apple cider vinegar or juice from half a lemon squeezed into it. You may also have one mug of organic black or green tea today.

Breakfast:
Morning Smoothie

Snack:
Bone Broth Egg Drop Soup
Liver Support Soup

Lunch:
Sweet Potato Toast with Mashed Avocado and grilled fish

Snack:
Golden Milk Bone Broth and simple sauerkraut

Dinner:
Vietnamese Spring Rolls
4 oz. bone broth of your choice

DAY SEVENTY-SEVEN (Phase 4; week 11)

Upon waking, make yourself a mug of fresh ginger tea with the juice from half a lemon squeezed into it *or* a mug of hot water with a shot of apple cider vinegar or juice from half a lemon squeezed into it. You may also have one mug of organic black or green tea today.

Breakfast:
Beth's Berry Brothie

Snack:
Butternut Squash Soup and simple sauerkraut
Liver Support Soup

Lunch:
Chicken and Asparagus Stir Fry (leftovers)

Snack:
Ginger Turmeric Bone Broth

Dinner:
Tuna Over Kale and a Sweet Potato (or leftover roasted veggies)
4 oz. Bone Broth of your choice

Phase 4 (week 12) Menu & Weekly Tips

Almost 80 days in! Can you feel all the cells in your body just buzzing with health and vitality?!?! I am just so proud of you for sticking to this plan. I hope by now you are seeing that way of living is going to give you so much more than better quality eggs and balanced hormones. Your body is cellularly different than it was just a few months ago *and* if you're like any of those subjects in the anti-aging research I discussed earlier in this book, you may now be 3 years YOUNGER on a physiological level than when you started this diet! WOW! That's amazing.

As a refresher, I want to remind you of the important daily tips you should still be doing each day on *The Egg Quality Diet:*

- Each day, be sure to drink about half your body weight in ounces of **filtered** water (keeping in mind not to force yourself to drink if you are not thirsty)
- Each serving size of protein (fish or meat) is 3 ounces or about the size of your palm. Your goal is 70-80 grams of protein per day or approximately 10-12 ounces of protein daily (see the Protein Cheat Sheet in the resources section for tips on achieving this)
- Each serving size of vegetable is ½ cup of cooked vegetables. Your goal is 6-8 servings (or 3-4 cups) of vegetables daily.
- It is important to keep your blood sugar balanced throughout your day, so do not go longer than 3-4 hours between eating meals/snacks
- If you have a known allergy to a certain food in the meal plan, please don't eat it
- If you get hungry, have ½ of a smoothie or grab an extra fat bomb or have some more carbohydrates in the form of sweet

potato or plantain chips or grab one of the On The Go snacks listed in your reference sheet

- If you're in doubt of your macronutrients, use the MyFitnessPal app to track them daily until you get into a rhythm reminder your goal is approximately 45% fat, 30% protein, and 25% carbs
- You'll notice we don't give exact measurements of food on the daily meal plans. Assume all serving sizes are 3-4 ounces (or the size of your palm) of proteins like meat and fish and that all vegetables are approximately 2-3 servings (1- 1 ½ cups of *cooked vegetables)* per meal or snack
- Keep it up with your regular servings of liver support soup. Ideally, you are having 4-6 ounces 5-7 times/week.
- Take time to meditate and/or journal each day about all the ways your body and your fertility is awakening. Head to AimeeRaupp.com/EQDiet for some of my guided meditations and mental/emotional exercises to get the most out of this plan.
- And, don't overlook the importance of sleep (it's ideal to get 7-8 hours nightly) and exercise (it's ideal to move your body 30-45 minutes 5-7 days/week).

Weekly Tip For Success:

This week, I think you are ready for another Story of Hope. In case you didn't know, every month on my social media channels I highlight a hopeful story from my clinic or online coaching program about a woman, just like you, who has finally gotten not only her BFP, but her baby (!!), after being on the fertility journey for too long. We have a lot of these stories highlighted for you on AimeeRaupp.com/EQDiet but I want to be sure you don't miss this one:

Story Of Hope: Janielle Was Told She Needed Donor Eggs To Get Pregnant https://youtu.be/Gk38TreZwcc

Your Mantra For The Week: I am allowed to have hope.

DAY SEVENTY-EIGHT (Phase 4; week 12)

Upon waking, make yourself a mug of fresh ginger tea with the juice from half a lemon squeezed into it *or* a mug of hot water with a shot of apple cider vinegar or juice from half a lemon squeezed into it. You may also have one mug of organic black or green tea today.

Breakfast:
Breakfast Hash and eggs

Snack:
Golden Milk Bone Broth with simple sauerkraut
Liver Support Soup

Lunch:
40 Clove Chicken and Sauteed Spinach

Snack:
Yolk Ocado

Dinner:
Spaghetti Zoodles with Faux-Mato Bolognese
4 oz. Bone Broth of your choice

DAY SEVENTY-NINE (Phase 4; week 12)

Upon waking, make yourself a mug of fresh ginger tea with the juice from half a lemon squeezed into it *or* a mug of hot water with a shot of apple cider vinegar or juice from half a lemon squeezed into it. You may also have one mug of organic black or green tea today.

Breakfast:
Sunrise Hash and eggs

Snack:
Butternut Squash Soup and simple sauerkraut
Liver Support Soup

Lunch:
Thai Crispy Pork Salad

Snack:
Ginger Turmeric Bone Broth

Dinner:
Grilled fish of choice with veggies
4 oz. Bone Broth of your choice

DAY EIGHTY (Phase 4; week 12)

Upon waking, make yourself a mug of fresh ginger tea with the juice from half a lemon squeezed into it *or* a mug of hot water with a shot of apple cider vinegar or juice from half a lemon squeezed into it. You may also have one mug of organic black or green tea today.

Breakfast:

Fruit Salad and a side of bacon

Snack:

Golden Milk Bone Broth and simple sauerkraut
Liver Support Soup

Lunch:

Zucchini Spinach Salad with Chicken

Snack:

Yolk Ocado

Dinner:

White Fish Packets with Zucchini and Summer Herbs
4 oz. Bone Broth of your choice

DAY EIGHTY-ONE (Phase 4; week 12)

Upon waking, make yourself a mug of fresh ginger tea with the juice from half a lemon squeezed into it *or* a mug of hot water with a shot of apple cider vinegar or juice from half a lemon squeezed into it. You may also have one mug of organic black or green tea today.

Breakfast:
Coconut Yogurt with cinnamon and fruit

Snack:
Bone Broth Egg Drop Soup and simple sauerkraut
Liver Support Soup

Lunch:
Sweet Potato Toast with mashed avocado and grilled fish of choice

Snack:
Matcha Latte and coconut yogurt

Dinner:
Grilled Sole with Asparagus and Broccoli sauteed in ghee
4 oz. Bone Broth of your choice

DAY EIGHTY-TWO (Phase 4; week 12)

Upon waking, make yourself a mug of fresh ginger tea with the juice from half a lemon squeezed into it *or* a mug of hot water with a shot of apple cider vinegar or juice from half a lemon squeezed into it. You may also have one mug of organic black or green tea today.

Breakfast:
Sunrise Hash and kombucha

Snack:
Yolk Ocado
Liver Support Soup

Lunch:
Grilled fish of choice with sauteed spinach and kale

Snack:
½ c. simple sauerkraut and a sweet potato with cultured ghee

Dinner:
Zucchini Spinach Salad with Chicken
4 oz. Bone Broth of your choice

DAY EIGHTY-THREE (Phase 4; week 12)

Upon waking, make yourself a mug of fresh ginger tea with the juice from half a lemon squeezed into it *or* a mug of hot water with a shot of apple cider vinegar or juice from half a lemon squeezed into it. You may also have one mug of organic black or green tea today.

Breakfast:
Mango Mint Smoothie

Snack:
Bone Broth Egg Drop Soup
Liver Support Soup

Lunch:
Sweet Potato Toast with Mashed Avocado and grilled fish of choice

Snack:
Golden Milk Bone Broth and simple sauerkraut

Dinner:
Whitefish Packets with Zucchini
4 oz. bone broth of your choice

DAY EIGHTY-FOUR (Phase 4; week 12)

Upon waking, make yourself a mug of fresh ginger tea with the juice from half a lemon squeezed into it *or* a mug of hot water with a shot of apple cider vinegar or juice from half a lemon squeezed into it. You may also have one mug of organic black or green tea today.

Breakfast:
Phase 2 Smoothie

Snack:
Butternut Squash Soup and simple sauerkraut
Liver Support Soup

Lunch:
Turkey and Bacon Roll-Ups with Radish Salad

Snack:
Ginger Turmeric Bone Broth

Dinner:
Ginger Lime Salmon Bowls
4 oz. Bone Broth of your choice and one egg yolk

Phase 4 (week 13) Menu & Weekly Tips

Are you still taking all of this in? Are you seeing the benefits of this life in your monthly menstrual cycle? Or better yet, did you fall pregnant yet? Or finally, have that IVF with good results? If so, make sure you share it with me and my team! We'd love to hear about all the changes you are seeing in your body and your fertility. And, even if you're not yet overflowing with pregnancy, know that you are doing so many beautiful things to support and nourish your body and you should be proud of yourself. Keep at it, your body is flourishing! P.S. make sure you're executing your daily tips as listed on page 182.

Weekly Tip For Success:
This week I want to talk to you about another kind of inflammation that could be dramatically impacting your health and fertility: emotional inflammation. Yes, the diet you are following is all about reducing inflammation in your body so that we can revitalize your egg quality. But, another major component of inflammation in your body includes the thoughts you think. As some of you may know, I have written a lot on this subject and I feel it is imperative to address it. So below you will see some of my favorite educational materials on managing emotional inflammation(reminder, all of these tools are also linked out on AimeeRaupp.com/EQDiet):

Is Fear Keeping You From Your Baby:
https://youtu.be/jUDt8SqURm0

This Kind Of Inflammation Is Affecting Your Egg Quality:
https://youtu.be/x3N-SCXrDeQ

Your Mantra For The Week: I am letting go of what no longer serves me.

DAY EIGHTY-FIVE (Phase 4; week 13)

Upon waking, make yourself a mug of fresh ginger tea with the juice from half a lemon squeezed into it *or* a mug of hot water with a shot of apple cider vinegar or juice from half a lemon squeezed into it. You may also have one mug of organic black or green tea today.

Breakfast:

Eggs and fruit salad

Snack:

Golden Milk Bone Broth and simple sauerkraut
Liver Support Soup

Lunch:

Butternut Squash Soup and grilled fish

Snack:

Yolk Ocado

Dinner:

Grilled fish and roasted veggies
4 oz. Bone Broth of your choice

DAY EIGHTY-SIX (Phase 4; week 13)

Upon waking, make yourself a mug of fresh ginger tea with the juice from half a lemon squeezed into it *or* a mug of hot water with a shot of apple cider vinegar or juice from half a lemon squeezed into it. You may also have one mug of organic black or green tea today.

Breakfast:
Maple Chicken Breakfast Sausage with Avocado

Snack:
Butternut Squash Soup and simple sauerkraut
Liver Support Soup

Lunch:
Mixed Veggie Noodles with Pork

Snack:
Ginger Turmeric Bone Broth

Dinner:
Pancit
4 oz. Bone Broth of your choice with one egg yolk

DAY EIGHTY-SEVEN (Phase 4; week 13)

Upon waking, make yourself a mug of fresh ginger tea with the juice from half a lemon squeezed into it *or* a mug of hot water with a shot of apple cider vinegar or juice from half a lemon squeezed into it. You may also have one mug of organic black or green tea today.

Breakfast:
Breakfast Hash and eggs

Snack:
Golden Milk Bone Broth
Liver Support Soup

Lunch:
Avocado Chicken Salad

Snack:
Yolk Ocado and simple sauerkraut

Dinner:
Grilled Sole with Asparagus and Hollandaise
4 oz. Bone Broth of your choice

DAY EIGHTY-EIGHT (Phase 4; week 13)

Upon waking, make yourself a mug of fresh ginger tea with the juice from half a lemon squeezed into it *or* a mug of hot water with a shot of apple cider vinegar or juice from half a lemon squeezed into it. You may also have one mug of organic black or green tea today.

Breakfast:
Sausage Patties, sauteed spinach, and mixed berries

Snack:
Bone Broth Egg Drop Soup and simple sauerkraut
Liver Support Soup

Lunch:
Sweet Potato Toast with Mashed Avocado and grilled fish

Snack:
Matcha Latte and coconut yogurt

Dinner:
Grilled fish of choice with roasted veggies
4 oz. Bone Broth of your choice

DAY EIGHTY-NINE (Phase 4; week 13)

Upon waking, make yourself a mug of fresh ginger tea with the juice from half a lemon squeezed into it *or* a mug of hot water with a shot of apple cider vinegar or juice from half a lemon squeezed into it. You may also have one mug of organic black or green tea today.

Breakfast:
Maple Chicken Breakfast Sausage with Avocado and mixed berries

Snack:
Yolk Ocado
Liver Support Soup

Lunch:
Vietnamese Spring Rolls and sauteed greens

Snack:
½ c. simple sauerkraut and a sweet potato with cultured ghee

Dinner:
Chinese Shredded Beef with Broccoli
4 oz. Bone Broth of your choice

DAY NINETY (Phase 4; week 13)

Upon waking, make yourself a mug of fresh ginger tea with the juice from half a lemon squeezed into it *or* a mug of hot water with a shot of apple cider vinegar or juice from half a lemon squeezed into it. You may also have one mug of organic black or green tea today.

Breakfast:
Breakfast Hash and eggs with mixed berries

Snack:
Bone Broth Egg Drop Soup and simple sauerkraut
Liver Support Soup

Lunch:
Grilled fish of choice with roasted veggies

Snack:
Golden Milk Bone Broth

Dinner:
Chicken, Broccoli, and Sweet Potato Sheet Pan Dinner
4 oz. bone broth of your choice

DAY NINETY-ONE (Phase 4; week 13)

Upon waking, make yourself a mug of fresh ginger tea with the juice from half a lemon squeezed into it *or* a mug of hot water with a shot of apple cider vinegar or juice from half a lemon squeezed into it. You may also have one mug of organic black or green tea today.

Breakfast:
Morning Smoothie

Snack:
Butternut Squash Soup and simple sauerkraut
Liver Support Soup

Lunch:
Chinese Shredded Beef with Broccoli

Snack:
Ginger Turmeric Bone Broth

Dinner:
Grilled fish of choice with sauteed greens
4 oz. Bone Broth of your choice

Phase 4 (week 14) Menu & Weekly Tips

You are officially in your last ten days of this meal plan. I am so excited for you! By now you should have reintroduced at least 2 dozen or so foods that you previously eliminated. And, it is my hope that through those introductions you learned a lot about your body. You are amazing and I hope you know that your insides are beaming with health and radiance. Your baby is so lucky to call the beautiful vessel that is your body its home. As we head to the end of this book, I encourage you to stay the course for the next 9 days as completing something you set out to do feels so damn good. And, don't forget to hit all your daily tips as mentioned on page 182.

Weekly Tip For Success:

For your last weekly tip, I want to talk about a very important topic: non-toxic bath, beauty, and household items. In this book, you learned all about how to heal your gut, balance hormones, and lower inflammation. Now (if you haven't already) it's time to take that level of healing to the superficial aspects of your body as the chemicals in your household products are major hormone disruptors that are wreaking havoc on your health and fertility. I cover this topic a lot on my social media platforms, but this video is one of my favorites on the topic. When you have time this week, watch it: https://www.youtube.com/watch?v=x5jD3gGY2iw&feature=yout u.be

Your Mantra For The Week: I am ready for the life of my dreams.

DAY NINETY-TWO (Phase 4; week 14)

Upon waking, make yourself a mug of fresh ginger tea with the juice from half a lemon squeezed into it *or* a mug of hot water with a shot of apple cider vinegar or juice from half a lemon squeezed into it. You may also have one mug of organic black or green tea today.

Breakfast:
Coconut Milk Yogurt with cinnamon and mixed berries

Snack:
Red Beet and Apple Salad

Lunch:
Sweet Potato Toast with mashed avocado and grilled fish of choice
Liver Support Soup

Snack:
Bone Broth Egg Drop Soup and simple sauerkraut

Dinner:
Shrimp Scampi with zoodles
4 oz. Bone Broth of your choice

DAY NINETY-THREE (Phase 4; week 14)

Upon waking, make yourself a mug of fresh ginger tea with the juice from half a lemon squeezed into it *or* a mug of hot water with a shot of apple cider vinegar or juice from half a lemon squeezed into it. You may also have one mug of organic black or green tea today.

Breakfast:
Sunrise Hash and eggs

Snack:
Ginger Turmeric Bone Broth

Lunch:
Grilled Cod with sauteed asparagus and leeks and hollandaise sauce
Liver Support Soup

Snack:
½ c. simple sauerkraut and a sweet potato with cultured ghee

Dinner:
Veggie Stir Fry with Shrimp
4 oz. Bone Broth of your choice

DAY NINETY-FOUR (Phase 4; week 14)

Upon waking, make yourself a mug of fresh ginger tea with the juice from half a lemon squeezed into it *or* a mug of hot water with a shot of apple cider vinegar or juice from half a lemon squeezed into it. You may also have one mug of organic black or green tea today.

Breakfast:
Plantain Waffles (freeze leftovers for next week) and side of berries

Snack:
Butternut Squash Soup and simple sauerkraut
Liver Support Soup

Lunch:
Vietnamese Spring Rolls and Broccoli Salad with Cranberries

Snack:
Ginger Turmeric Bone Broth

Dinner:
Beef Barbacoa Bowls (reserve extra beef for tomorrow night, no need to freeze)
4 oz. Bone Broth of your choice

DAY NINETY-FIVE (Phase 4; week 14)

Upon waking, make yourself a mug of fresh ginger tea with the juice from half a lemon squeezed into it *or* a mug of hot water with a shot of apple cider vinegar or juice from half a lemon squeezed into it. You may also have one mug of organic black or green tea today.

Breakfast:
Maple Chicken Breakfast Sausage and Avocado

Snack:
Golden Milk Bone Broth and simple sauerkraut
Liver Support Soup

Lunch:
Stir Fried Greens with Sausage and Roasted Beets

Snack:
Yolk Ocado

Dinner:
Shredded Beef Tacos with Mango Salsa and Roasted Root Veggies (use extra beef from the previous night)
4 oz. Bone Broth of your choice

DAY NINETY-SIX (Phase 4; week 14)

Upon waking, make yourself a mug of fresh ginger tea with the juice from half a lemon squeezed into it *or* a mug of hot water with a shot of apple cider vinegar or juice from half a lemon squeezed into it. You may also have one mug of organic black or green tea today.

Breakfast:
Fruit Salad and Bacon (throw together your favorite fruit and your favorite bacon, easy peasy)

Snack:
Bone Broth Egg Drop Soup and simple sauerkraut
Liver Support Soup

Lunch:
Sweet Potato Toast with mashed avocado and grilled fish of choice

Snack:
Matcha Latte and coconut yogurt

Dinner:
Slow Cooker Ham (takes six hours on low- plan ahead) and leftover Roasted Root Veggies
4 oz. Bone Broth of your choice

DAY NINETY-SEVEN (Phase 4; week 14)

Upon waking, make yourself a mug of fresh ginger tea with the juice from half a lemon squeezed into it *or* a mug of hot water with a shot of apple cider vinegar or juice from half a lemon squeezed into it. You may also have one mug of organic black or green tea today.

Breakfast:
Ham and Eggs (warm some leftover ham from last night and prepare eggs however you'd like)

Snack:
Yolk Ocado
Liver Support Soup

Lunch:
Sweet potato and grilled fish of choice

Snack:
½ c. simple sauerkraut and a sweet potato with cultured ghee

Dinner:
Grilled Cod with sauteed asparagus and leeks and hollandaise sauce
4 oz. Bone Broth of your choice

DAY NINETY-EIGHT (Phase 4; week 14)

Upon waking, make yourself a mug of fresh ginger tea with the juice from half a lemon squeezed into it *or* a mug of hot water with a shot of apple cider vinegar or juice from half a lemon squeezed into it. You may also have one mug of organic black or green tea today.

Breakfast:
Garden Green Brothie

Snack:
Bone Broth Egg Drop Soup
Liver Support Soup

Lunch:
Sweet Potato Toast with Mashed Avocado and 4 oz. bone broth of your choice

Snack:
Golden Milk Bone Broth

Dinner:
Vietnamese Spring Rolls and Broccoli Salad with Cranberries (leftover from earlier in the week)
4 oz. bone broth of your choice

DAY NINETY-NINE (Phase 4; week 15)

Upon waking, make yourself a mug of fresh ginger tea with the juice from half a lemon squeezed into it *or* a mug of hot water with a shot of apple cider vinegar or juice from half a lemon squeezed into it. You may also have one mug of organic black or green tea today.

Breakfast:
Maple Chicken Sausage and eggs with Fruit Salad

Snack:
Butternut Squash Soup
Liver Support Soup

Lunch:
Grilled Fish with sauteed greens and simple sauerkraut

Snack:
Ginger Turmeric Bone Broth

Dinner:
Shredded Beef Tacos with Mango Salsa and Roasted Root Veggies
4 oz. Bone Broth of your choice

DAY ONE HUNDRED (Phase 4; week 15)

Upon waking, make yourself a mug of fresh ginger tea with the juice from half a lemon squeezed into it *or* a mug of hot water with a shot of apple cider vinegar or juice from half a lemon squeezed into it. You may also have one mug of organic black or green tea today.

Breakfast:

Plantain Waffles and fruit salad

Snack:

Butternut Squash Soup
Liver Support Soup

Lunch:

Turkey and Bacon Roll-Ups with Radish Salad

Snack:

Ginger Turmeric Bone Broth and simple sauerkraut

Dinner:

40 Clove Chicken and spinach sauteed in ghee (no need to freeze extra chicken, you're using it tomorrow)
4 oz. Bone Broth of your choice

CHAPTER SEVEN

Beyond The 100 Days Of
The Egg Quality Diet

You did it! You made it through 100 days of one of the most powerfully anti-aging, egg quality improving eating plans that exists. I hope you are feeling amazingly renewed and full of hope. At this point in *The Egg Quality Diet,* you have figured out exactly what foods work for your body and which ones don't. And, that is how I want you to live-- what that knowledge in mind. You now have your very own roadmap to what truly nourishes the cells in your body and it is my belief that you are closer than ever to creating that dream baby. Now, your only job is to continue to show up for your body the way you did the past 100 days. Keeping in mind what you learned about your body and the nourishment it needs. Let the kinks in your system be your guide. Let the plentiful resources found on AimeeRaupp.com/EQDiet support all the ways you can maximize your fertility. And, let the hope in your heart be your beacon. Know that as you continue to feed your body this way, your gut will continue to heal, your inflammation will continue to dissipate and your body will be prepared to get and stay pregnant. If you happen to deviate from this style of living and eating, be easy on yourself and know that you can always return to it. Sometimes I go back and do a few days in Phase 2 to 'reset' my body if I feel the need to.

As I said at the beginning of this book, I can't promise you when this baby is going to come through but what I can promise you is that your body is more prepared now than ever before to receive this child. So, as I say to my clients all the time: you remain here, in your preparedness for this child to come through and allow the rest to unfold. I know the waiting is grueling and truly the hardest part on this journey so continue to use the mindset tools I have for you on the website that accompanies this book, stay open in your heart, and be proud of yourself for how you are showing up for you. Through these past 100 days, you have learned how to nourish and mother yourself and with that, you are solid in your readiness to be the kind of mother you have always dreamed of being. I am steadfastly cheering you on. Continue to follow me on all my social channels so that I may continue to inspire you on this journey.

All my love to you and your growing family,

Aimee

Weekly Shopping Lists

WEEK 1 SHOPPING LIST (Phase 1)
(this shopping list is also available for download on AimeeRaupp.com/EQDiet)

You're only going to need one cup of bone broth this week (at the very end of the week). Sometime during the week make your first batch of bone broth and freeze it for next week (see simple bone broth recipe at the back of this book or visit AimeeRaupp.com/EQDiet for approved store-bought/packaged broths). Soon making your bone broth will be routine.

You may have some of these items in your cupboards already, if so, cross them off your list!

Assume that all items on the list are organic, grass-fed, pastured, and non-genetically modified (excluding vegetables on the clean 15 list at the back of this book (as well this list is on AimeeRaupp.com/EQDiet) as the clean 15 veggies don't need to be organic

Pantry Staples:

- One bottle of apple cider vinegar (the real stuff with the mother)
- Vital Proteins Beef Gelatin
- Vital Proteins Collagen Peptides
- Extra virgin, cold-pressed olive oil
- Extra virgin, cold-pressed coconut oil
- Pink Himalayan sea salt
- Black pepper
- Arrowroot
- Maple Syrup
- Garlic powder

- Cultured Ghee (I recommend the brand Pure Indian)

Produce

- Fresh cilantro (1 bunch)
- Fresh parsley (2 bunches)
- Fresh basil (1 bunch)
- Fresh rosemary (1 bunch)
- 2 bulbs of garlic
- 3 tomatoes
- Spinach (2 packages)
- 5 avocados
- 3 lemons
- 1 lime
- 3 sweet potatoes
- Blueberries (2 cups)
- Mesclun greens (1 package)
- Mixed greens (1 package)
- Green beans
- Olives
- Banana (1)
- Green apple (1)
- Kale (2 bunches)
- Celery (2 heads)
- Beets (3)
- Golden beet (1)
- Parsnip (1)
- White sweet potato (1)
- Cauliflower (1 head)
- Bok choy
- Strawberries (1 package)
- Carrots (1 package- whole)

- Shallot (1)
- Yellow onion (3)
- Green onion (1)
- Mushrooms (shiitake or maitake)
- Mushrooms (cremini)
- Leeks
- Asparagus (2 bunches)
- Grapefruit (2)
- Cabbage, red or green- 4-5 heads (*this is for making sauerkraut, if you do not wish to make your own sauerkraut please skip this*)
- Romaine (1 head)
- Broccoli (2 heads)
- Green plantain (2)

Proteins

- 1 package grass-fed, gluten-free sausages (chicken, pork, or beef)
- 1 dozen pastured eggs
- Bacon (nitrate free) (6 slices)
- 1 lb Wild salmon
- 1 ¼ chicken breast
- ⅓ - ½ lb. Beef tenderloin
- ¾ lb. ribeye steak
- 6 oz. Sole
- 1 whole free-range chicken or 2 to 3 pounds of bony chicken parts, such as necks, backs, breastbones, and wings (or beef bones)
- 2-4 chicken feet

Other Items

- 1 can full-fat coconut milk (in BPA free cans, I like the brand Native Forest of 365)
- 1 coconut milk yogurt (free of additives and added sugar, I like the brand Anita's)
- 2 LaraBars
- 2 Epic Bison Cranberry bars
- Hummus
- 1 package quinoa or brown rice pasta
- Almond butter *(if you already have nut butter in your pantry just use whatever you have since we'll be eliminating this after the Phase 1 Phase)*
- 1-2 cups Almonds *(if you already have nuts in your pantry just use whatever you have since we'll be eliminating these after the Phase 1 Phase)*

Week 2 SHOPPING LIST
(partial Phase 1 & Phase 2)
(this list is also available for download on
AimeeRaupp.com/EQDiet)

You're going to need at least 18 cups of bone broth this week. You already made and froze your first batch so you're set for a few days. Sometime during the week make your second batch of bone broth and freeze it for the rest of the week.

You may have some of these items in your cupboards already, if so, cross them off your list!

Remember you can also purchase pre-made bone broth that is Aimee Approved at AimeeRaupp.com/BoneBroth

Assume that all items on the list are organic, grass-fed, pastured, and non-GM (excluding vegetables on the clean 15 list as these veggies don't need to be organic).

Pantry Staples *(buy these once and you'll be set for the rest of the program)*:

- Bone Broth Protein
- Coconut flour *(keep in mind, after Phase 1 is complete you are NOT consuming any flours again for several weeks)*
- Oregano
- Bay leaves
- Ground turmeric
- Ground ginger
- Ground cinnamon
- Ground coriander
- Ground cumin
- Mustard seed
- Probiotic (for making coconut yogurt)

Produce

- Fresh cilantro (1 bunch)
- Fresh parsley (1 bunch)
- Fresh basil (1 bunch)
- Fresh ginger
- 1 bulb of garlic
- Spinach (3-4 packages)
- Kale (1 package)
- Dandelion greens
- Asparagus (1 bunch)
- 5 avocados
- 8 lemons
- 4 limes
- 4 sweet potatoes
- 2 plantains
- 1 banana
- Berries of your choice (2 cups)
- Capers
- Olives, green pitted
- Swiss chard (1 bunch)
- Broccoli (1 head)
- Cauliflower (1 head)
- 3 Green onions
- 3 yellow onions
- Shiitake mushrooms
- 10 beets
- 10 carrots
- Celery (1 head)
- 32 oz. butternut squash

Proteins

- 4 Eggs
- 1 lb. boneless, skinless chicken thighs
- ½ lb. wild shrimp
- 1 lb. Salmon
- 6 oz. steak
- 1 lb. wild cod
- 1 lb. lamb
- 4-5 lbs. Bones (for broth)
- 1-2 chicken feet (for broth)

Other

- 1 EPIC Bison Cranberry Bar
- 1 bottle kombucha *(less than 5g sugar per serving)*
- Shredded coconut
- 1 can/box coconut cream/coconut butter
- Fish sauce
- 6 cans coconut milk, full fat

WEEK THREE SHOPPING LIST (Phase 2)

(this shopping list is also available for download on AimeeRaupp.com/EQDiet)

You're going to need at least 20 cups of bone broth this week. Early this week make two batches of bone broth (or split it up throughout the week) and freeze so you can pull out just what you'll need the day before.

You may have some of these items in your cupboards already, if so, cross them off your list!

Remember you can also purchase pre-made bone broth that is Aimee Approved at AimeeRaupp.com/BoneBroth

Assume that all items on the list are organic, grass-fed, pastured, and non-GM (excluding vegetables on the clean 15 list as these veggies don't need to be organic).

Pantry Staples *(buy these once and you'll be set for the rest of the program)*:

- Basil
- Oregano
- Thyme
- Marjoram

Produce

- Fresh cilantro (1 bunch)
- Fresh parsley (1 bunch)
- Fresh ginger
- 1 bulb of garlic
- Spinach (3 packages)
- Kale (1 package)
- Dandelion greens
- Asparagus (1 bunch)

- 5 avocados
- 8 lemons
- 6 sweet potatoes
- 20 Olives, kalamata pitted
- Broccoli (1 head)
- Cauliflower (1 head)
- Scallions (1 bunch)
- 3 yellow onions
- 10 beets
- 2 lb. carrots
- Celery (2 heads)
- 2 zucchini
- 1 banana

Proteins

- 5 Eggs
- 1/2 lb. Salmon
- 6 oz. steak
- 1 lb. wild cod
- 1 lb. lamb
- 8-10 lbs. Bones (for broth)
- 4 chicken feet (for broth)

Other

- 1 bottle kombucha
- 4 cans coconut milk, full fat

WEEK FOUR SHOPPING LIST (Phase 3)

(this shopping list is also available for download on AimeeRaupp.com/EQDiet)

You're going to need at least 30 cups of bone broth this week. Early this week make three batches of bone broth (or split it up throughout the week) and freeze so you can pull out just what you'll need the day before. Or purchase approved bone broth at AimeeRaupp.com/BoneBroth

You may have some of these items in your cupboards already, if so, cross them off your list!

Assume that all items on the list are organic, grass-fed, pastured, and non-GM (excluding vegetables on the clean 15 list (https://www.ewg.org/foodnews/clean-fifteen.php) as these veggies don't need to be organic).

Produce

- Fresh cilantro (1 bunch)
- Fresh parsley (2-3 bunches)
- Fresh oregano
- Fresh ginger
- 2 bulbs of garlic
- Spinach (2 packages)
- Kale (1 package)
- Arugula (1 package)
- Dandelion greens
- Asparagus (2 bunches)
- 6 avocados
- 10 lemons
- 10 limes
- 3 sweet potatoes
- 4 white sweet potatoes
- Broccoli (1 head)

- Cauliflower (2 heads)
- Scallions (1 bunch)
- 3 yellow onions
- 1 red onion
- 7 beets
- 1 golden beet
- 1 parsnip
- 1 bok choy
- 2 leeks
- 2 lb. carrots
- Celery (2 heads)
- 8 zucchini
- 2 banana
- 1 grapefruit
- 1 large or 2 small mangoes
- Red grapes
- 4 red apples
- 1 green apple
- 4 lbs butternut squash
- 1 head cabbage
- 3 stalks lemongrass
- Mint
- 1 spaghetti squash
- 2 lbs mushrooms

Proteins

- 12 Eggs
- 4 chicken breast
- 1/2 lb. Salmon
- 6 oz. steak
- 1/2 lb. wild cod

- 2 c. ham
- 1 ½ lb. ground pork
- 2 ¾ lb. shrimp
- 2 c. shredded pork
- 12 brats (or any AIP friendly mild sausage)
- 1 lb. bacon (AIP friendly)
- 8-10 lbs. Bones (for broth)
- 4 chicken feet (for broth)

Other

- 7 cans coconut milk, full fat
- Coconut flakes (1 package)

SHOPPING LIST TEMPLATE
(Phase 3 & 4)
(this shopping list is also available for download on AimeeRaupp.com/EQDiet)

This list is your template for going forward. It includes the ingredients for bone broth plus proteins, plenty of veggies, Liver Support Juice, pantry staples, and On The Go Snacks. Feel free to switch it up and add to it as you meal plan and customize The Egg Quality Diet to your needs.

You may have some of these items in your cupboards already, if so, cross them off your list!

Remember you can also purchase pre-made bone broth that is Aimee Approved at AimeeRaupp.com/BoneBroth

Assume that all items on the list are organic, grass-fed, pastured, and non-GM (excluding vegetables on the clean 15 list (link to: https://www.ewg.org/foodnews/clean-fifteen.php) as these veggies don't need to be organic).

Pantry Staples:

- One bottle of apple cider vinegar (the real stuff with the mother)
- Vital Proteins Beef Gelatin
- Vital Proteins Collagen Peptides
- Bone broth protein powder
- Extra virgin, cold-pressed olive oil
- Extra virgin, cold-pressed coconut oil
- Pink Himalayan sea salt
- Organic Ghee (I recommend the brand, Pure Indian)

Produce

- Fresh cilantro (1 bunch)
- Fresh parsley (2 bunches)
- Fresh basil (1 bunch)
- Fresh rosemary (1 bunch)
- 2 bulbs of garlic
- Spinach (2 packages)
- avocados
- lemons
- sweet potatoes
- Mesclun greens (1 package)
- Mixed greens (1 package)
- Green beans
- Kale (2 bunches)
- Celery (2 heads)
- Beets
- Cauliflower
- Bok choy
- Carrots (1 package- whole)
- Yellow onion (3)
- Green onion (1)
- Asparagus (2 bunches)
- Broccoli (2 heads)
- Green plantain (2)

Proteins

- 1 package grass-fed, gluten-free sausages (chicken, pork, or beef); make sure these are free of nightshade vegetables, nuts, and seeds depending on where you are with reintroductions
- 1 dozen pastured eggs
- Bacon (nitrate-free)

- 1 lb Wild salmon
- chicken breast or thighs chicken breast
- Beef tenderloin
- ¾ lb. ribeye steak
- Sole or any other wild-caught fish you prefer (don't forget to check out https://www.seafoodwatch.org/ for best seafood choices in your area)
- 1 lb. ground lamb or turkey
- 1 whole free-range chicken or 2 to 3 pounds of bony chicken parts, such as necks, backs, breastbones, and wings (or beef bones)
- 2-4 chicken feet
- Any other protein you choose that is acceptable for this eating plan

Other Items

- 1 can full-fat coconut milk (in BPA free cans, I like the brands Native Forest or 365)
- 1 coconut milk yogurt (free of additives and added sugar, I like the brand Anita's)

On The Go Snacks (approved for Phase 3 & 4)

I know how hectic life can be, so I went ahead and gathered some easy on-the-go snacks for you that can be store-bought. As of when I wrote this book (April 2021), these snacks and brands are all approved for Phase 3 & Phase 4 of The Egg Quality Diet, but always read ingredients to be certain:

- Epic Cranberry Bison Bars
- Organic Gemeni Raw Tiger Nuts
- Artisana Coconut Butter

- Bare Simply Cinnamon Organic Apple Chips
- Dang Lightly Salted Toasted Coconut Chips
- Nutiva Coconut Manna
- Jackson's Honest Sweet Potato Chips
- Freeze Dried Blueberries
- SeaSnax
- Wild Planet Wild Alaskan Salmon
- Wild Planet Sardines
- Organic Apple Butter
- Pork Clouds Rosemary & Sea Salt Pork Rinds
- Paleo Angel Power Balls
- Yucan Crunch
- Wild Zora Lamb & Veggie Jerky
- Pure Traditions Cranberry Beef & Organ Strips
- Barnana Organic Plantain Chips
- Anita's Plain Coconut Milk Yogurt
- GT's Kombucha (just watch the sugar content on any kombucha you consume)
- Trader Joe's Organic Coconut Smoothie

If/when you have successfully reintroduced nuts and seeds, here are some other on the go snack ideas:

- Kit's Organic Bars
- Lara Bars
- RX Bars
- Artisana Nut Butter packets
- Basilicotta Nut "Cheese" spread
- Treeline nut cheese spread

keep in mind you will likely be able to find all of these products on Amazon.com

Resources

In this section I have gathered information on two potential issues that may be the cause of you not feeling as good as you should be on The Egg Quality Diet. I urge you to read through both the histamine and SIBO information on the pages that follow and adopt my recommendations. As well, check out the resources listed for you on AimeeRaupp.com/EQDiet as that is where you will find educational tools, videos, further reading, supplement recommendations, and more.

Is Too Much Histamine Affecting Your Health and Your Fertility?

Histamine isn't a bad thing. In fact, it's something we need for a normally functioning immune system. Histamine is a normal biochemical produced by immune cells during certain immune responses that produce some unpleasant but necessary effects. Think stuffy nose from seasonal allergies or challenges breathing when we get hives or the red raised bumps that happen after a mosquito bite. Histamine is also responsible for promoting gastric acid secretion and has a regulatory effect on neurotransmitters. The issue with histamine is when your body can't break it down fast enough or you simply make too much. My recommendation is that if you see yourself in some or many of the below symptoms AND you are having challenges getting pregnant, then I want you to adopt a low-histamine diet for at least one month. Once your symptoms begin shifting, then you can SLOWLY add back in some of the higher histamine foods and see how your body reacts. If your symptom reappears then you must continue to eliminate that food.

Symptoms of high histamine levels in your body:

- Headaches/migraines
- Difficulty falling asleep, easily arousal
- Hypertension (high blood pressure)
- Vertigo or dizziness
- Arrhythmia, or accelerated heart rate
- Difficulty regulating body temperature
- Anxiety
- Nausea and/or vomiting
- Abdominal cramps
- Facial flushing
- Nasal congestion, sneezing, difficulty breathing
- Abnormal menstrual cycle
- Rosacea
- Eczema or Psoriasis
- Hives or itchy, rashy skin
- Fatigue
- Tissue swelling

You can have high histamine levels for a couple of reasons:

Bad gut bacteria: Many gut bacteria produce histamine themselves. If these histamine-producing strains are overrepresented in your gut, you may suffer negative symptoms from any extra histamine.

Mast cell activation syndrome: Mast cells are immune cells that produce histamine as part of the immune response. There is a newly identified health issue called mast cell activation syndrome (MCAS) where a person's mast cells release excessive amounts of histamine.

And, there are a few more reasons why we can't break down the high levels of histamine:

Bad gut bacteria: Many gut bacteria also degrade histamine. A dearth of these histamine-degrading strains in the gut may lead to impaired histamine degradation and increased histamine load.

Diamine oxidase deficiency: Some histamine intolerance stems from a simple deficiency in diamine oxidase, the enzyme that breaks down histamine in the body. Without adequate diamine oxidase, histamine builds up and causes problems where it shouldn't.

HNMT deficiency: We produce another histamine-degrading enzyme called HNMT, or histamine N-methyltransferase. HNMT deficiency is largely genetic, as various HNMT polymorphisms determine endogenous histamine levels.

The Low- Histamine Diet

This list may contain a lot of foods you consume on a regular basis. You can't avoid all histamines as they are a naturally occurring substances. But you can consume fewer histamines on a daily basis. So it's not about complete elimination of all these foods, it's about frequency and consistency when ingesting high histamine foods. I recommend you minimize exposure and aim for 3-5 servings per week of these foods, or if you notice a clear-cut reaction from one of these foods, then avoid altogether.

Foods to avoid/have in moderation:

- Shellfish or fin fish, fresh, frozen, smoked, or canned
- Processed, cured, smoked, and fermented meats such as lunch meat, bacon, sausage, salami, pepperoni
- Leftover meat (After meat is cooked, the histamine levels increase due to microbial action as the meat sits). Don't eat meat that's refrigerated for more than 2 days after it's been cooked. *This is not a food I want you avoiding, rather I recommend cooking fresh meat and consuming it that day or the next.*
- Leftover bone broth (similar to meat, don't consume bone broth that's refrigerated for more than 2 days after it's been cooked/defrosted) *This is not a food I want you avoiding, rather I recommend cooking your broth for less time on the stovetop (8 hours or less) or cook it in the instant pot AND freeze in small batches. Thaw a new batch daily for consumption that day or the next.*
- All fermented milk products, including most cheeses
- Yogurt, buttermilk, kefir
- Citrus fruits – eg. oranges, grapefruit, lemons, lime
- Nuts- namely cashews, walnuts, and peanuts (but I find that too many almonds can also aggravate my eczema, so I would tune in and pay attention to how your body reacts to all nuts as recommended in my diet plan)
- Blackberries and strawberries
- Dried fruit
- Fermented foods: sauerkraut, kombucha, pickles, relishes, fermented soy products (Fermented foods are some of the biggest culprits since even beneficial bacteria produce histamine during fermentation. In fact, reacting to fermented

foods is a classic sign of histamine intolerance, especially if probiotic supplements are well-tolerated.)

- Spinach *This is not a food I want you avoiding (unless you have a clear reaction/allergy), rather I recommend consuming in moderation, about 3-5 servings/week.*
- Avocado *This is not a food I want you avoiding (unless you have a clear reaction/allergy), rather I recommend consuming in moderation, about 3-5 servings/week.*
- Beans
- Tomatoes- including ketchup, tomato sauces
- Artificial food colors and preservatives
- Spices: cinnamon, chili powder, cloves, anise, nutmeg, curry powder, cayenne
- Alcohol
- Chocolate, cocoa
- Vinegar and foods containing vinegar such as pickles, relishes, ketchup, and prepared mustard

For more resources, check out The Low Histamine Chef (aka Yasmina Ykelenstam). As well as this informative histamine intolerance food list.

Low Histamine Foods THAT YOU CAN EAT:

- Fresh meat (cooled, frozen, or fresh)
- Freshly caught fish
- Chicken (skinned and fresh)
- Egg yolk
- Fresh fruits – with the exception of strawberries and blackberries, most fresh fruits are considered to have a low histamine level (also see histamine liberators below)
- Fresh vegetables – with the exception of tomatoes

- Grains – rice noodles, yeast-free rye bread, rice crisp bread, oats, puffed rice crackers, millet flour, pasta (spelt and corn-based)
- Milk substitutes – coconut milk, rice milk
- Bone broth that is cooked on the stovetop for less than 8 hours, or in the instant pot for 2 hours. Freeze in small batches for daily consumption. If you have a histamine issue it is highly recommended to consume freshly made bone broth or broth that has been thawed that same day. Broth left in the refrigerator for more than 1 day will have high histamine levels.
- Grass-Fed butter and/or ghee (choose ghee if you're avoiding dairy)
- Coconut oil and/or olive oil
- Most leafy herbs
- Most non-citric fruit juices

A side note on healing your gut from a histamine excess:

While it's true that fermented foods are great for restoring normal gut flora, sauerkraut certainly isn't the be-all and end-all. A good probiotic supplement and a diet rich in prebiotic foods such as chicory root, artichokes, dandelion greens, garlic, leek, onion, and asparagus can be of assistance.

While probiotics such as Lactobacillus rhamnosus suppress histamine receptors, prebiotics are carbohydrates that are indigestible for humans but that act as a food source for beneficial bacteria (the probiotics). Nigella sativa or black cumin is a spice that has been used in Ayurvedic medicine for centuries and has recently shown promise as a natural antihistamine for treating seasonal allergies.

DAO supplements are also available. However, these have had mixed results and come with a hefty price tag making them a poor choice for long-term treatment. You can also make certain dietary changes to improve your symptoms. Vitamin B6, copper, and Vitamin C are DAO cofactors, so make sure your diet is rich in these nutrients. D-Hist by Ortho Molecular is a great multi-faceted product that addresses many histamine issues. Head to AimeeRaupp.com/EQDiet for a list of all my recommended supplements for fertility.

Vitamin B6 can be found in chicken, turkey, and potatoes. Liver and asparagus are rich sources of copper, and finally vitamin C can be found in all fruits and vegetables, particularly in kiwifruit, oranges, and berries.

As with any food elimination diet, there's no point in following something when you know in your gut (excuse the pun) that it isn't helping. Nevertheless, if your dietary attempts to date have failed then there is no harm in temporarily trying out a low histamine diet to see if it works for you.

Is Small Intestine Bacterial Overgrowth (SIBO) Affecting Your Health & Fertility?

Small intestinal bacterial overgrowth (SIBO) occurs when there is an abnormal increase in the overall bacterial population in the small intestine, the part of the gut that connects the stomach to the large intestine. The small intestine is where most of your nutrients are absorbed and although it is normal to have some bacteria there, most of it should be in the large intestine, *not the small intestine.* SIBO commonly results when the passage of food and waste products in the digestive tract is slowed down, creating a breeding ground for bacteria. The excess bacteria often cause digestive disturbances like:

- bloating (to the point where you look pregnant) especially after eating and above your belly button
- A very fast feeling of fullness when you start eating
- Excessive belching A feeling of slow digestion
- Food intolerances
- Excessive (and stinky) gas even after eating healthy foods
- Diarrhea or oily looking bowel movements
- Abdominal discomfort, cramping, or pain
- Nausea

According to Aviva Romm, M.D., "Digestion and the maintenance of healthy gut flora rely on a delicate orchestration, from mouth to opposite end, of enzymes, hormones, nerves and muscles that break our food down and move nutrients and waste through the digestive tract. SIBO is sometimes caused by serious or permanent conditions like scarring or strictures in the digestive tract from Crohn's disease, radiation, or surgery, or small intestinal diverticulosis, or motility problems from nerve damage, scleroderma, or diabetes. However, it can also be caused by common medications and lifestyle habits that disrupt this balance, such as low stomach acid due to diet, age or antacid medication use, recent or frequent use of antibiotics throughout your life affecting healthy gut flora, stress affecting gut motility, blood flow to the gut walls, and digestion – all of which can be improved."

If you suspect you have SIBO, you can get tested. The most common test is a Breath Test which can be done by your functional medicine doctor or a gastrointestinal doctor.

To treat SIBO, you have to restore normal gut bacteria function. What many doctors have found is that the best way to do this is to follow a LOW FODMAP diet (more on that below) along with antibiotic treatment (rifaximin is the most commonly used one for SIBO) and/or herbal antibiotics like goldenseal, black walnut, oregano oil and more. If you suspect you have SIBO I highly recommend finding a healthcare practitioner to help you diagnose and treat it (Aviva Romm, Mark Hyman, Frank Lipman, and Chris Kresser all have great resources on their respective websites for how to best handle SIBO).

As SIBO pertains to *The Egg Quality Diet* I find that with a few LOW FODMAP tweaks you can start feeling better and continue healing your gut through this elimination protocol. The LOW FODMAP diet was designed by researchers at Monash University to improve IBS symptoms. The diet focuses on removing carbohydrates that are high in fermentable oligosaccharides, disaccharides, monosaccharides, and polyols. This diet is also used for SIBO because high FODMAP carbohydrate foods can ferment in the gut and feed a bacterial overgrowth. I find that when women who are experiencing SIBO symptoms (or know they have SIBO) avoid the following foods while doing *The Egg Quality Diet* they feel MUCH better:

- Artichokes
- Garlic
- Onion
- Onion and garlic powder
- Asparagus
- Beets

- Broccoli
- Brussel sprouts
- Cabbage
- Cauliflower
- Fennel
- Okra
- Mushrooms
- All peas, beans, and nightshade vegetables
- All fermented foods, including kombucha, vinegar, yogurt, sauerkraut, and kimchi

Also, pay attention to the high histamine food lists as mentioned on page 229.

RECIPES

40 Clove Chicken:

Adapted from Real Plans
Makes 4 Servings

Ingredients:

3 pounds whole chicken
2 heads garlic
2 tablespoons coconut oil
coarse sea salt, to taste
1/2 bunch chives, optional

Directions:

1. Preheat the oven to 375F.
2. Remove chicken from the package, remove giblet bag from the chicken cavity, rinse well, and pat dry. Save giblets in the fridge for making stock.
3. Separate and peel the garlic cloves. Soften coconut oil, if solid.
4. Rub the softened oil over chicken skin.
5. Sprinkle generously with sea salt.
6. Layer garlic in a baking dish and place the trussed and seasoned chicken on top of the garlic.
7. Bake for 30 minutes, then using tongs and/or potholders, gently flip the chicken so that the legs are up.
8. Salt the flip side of the chicken and bake for a total time of 20 minutes per pound. The chicken is done when a meat

thermometer inserted into the leg or inner thigh (avoiding the bone) reads 165F and the skin is nicely browned and crisp.

9. Mince chives.

10. Gently remove the chicken to a serving platter, serve with roasted garlic and sprinkled generously with fresh chives.

Arugula, Avocado, and Grapefruit Salad:

From Real Plans
makes 2 servings

Ingredients:

1/2 lemon

2 avocados

1 pink grapefruit

1/4 cup extra virgin olive oil

3/4 teaspoon coarse sea salt

2 handfuls of baby arugula

Directions:

1. Wash baby arugula, juice the lemon, and peel and cut avocados into ¾ chunks. Segment the grapefruits.
2. Place the olive oil, lemon juice, salt, into a small glass jar.
3. Secure the lid and shake well until dressing is well combined.
4. Toss the arugula in the dressing.
5. Top with the avocado chunks and grapefruit segments; serve.

Avocado Chicken Salad:

Adapted from Real Plans
makes 2 servings

Ingredients:

3/4 pound chicken breast (or leftover chicken from your bone broth, that's what I use)

1 tablespoon coconut oil

1 1/2 large avocados

1 green onion

1/4 bunch cilantro

1/2 lime

1/4 teaspoon garlic powder

1/2 teaspoon coarse sea salt, plus more to taste

4 ounces mixed greens

Directions:

1. In a skillet over medium-high heat, saute chicken in coconut oil until browned on the outside and cooked through. Set aside to cool.
2. Peel, pit, and chop avocado. Mince green onion and cilantro, and juice the lime. When the chicken is cooled, shred apart or dice into half-inch cubes.
3. Combine all ingredients (except salad greens) in a large bowl and mash with a fork to combine.
4. Season with additional sea salt to taste and serve over greens.

Beef Barbacoa Bowls (Instant Pot Recipe):

Adapted from Real Plans
Makes 4 Servings

Ingredients:

1/2 bunch cilantro

1/2 red onion

5 cloves garlic

1 lime

2 carrots

1/2 teaspoon ground cloves

1 1/2 teaspoons coarse sea salt

1/4 cup apple cider vinegar

1/4 cup filtered water, as needed

2 pounds beef brisket, or chuck roast

1 bay leaf

2 green onions

1 avocado

1/2 pound spinach

For the cauliflower rice:

1/2 head cauliflower

1 small onion

1 clove garlic

1 tablespoon coconut oil, or fat of your choice

2 teaspoons coarse sea salt

Directions:

1. Divide the cilantro. Peel and cut the red onion into large chunks.

2. Peel and smash the cloves of garlic. Juice the lime. Peel and coarsely chop the carrots.

3. In a food processor with the s-blade, pulse red onion, garlic, cloves, salt, lime juice, apple cider vinegar, and 1/2 of the cilantro until smooth. Add water, if needed, to ensure that you have at least 1/2 cup of sauce.

4. Add sauce to the pressure cooker and place the brisket on top of this mixture. Place chopped carrots and bay leaves on top.

5. Close lid and pressure cook for 45 minutes.

6. While meat is cooking, dice the green onions. Peel and slice the avocado. Steam the spinach.

7. When meat is done cooking, release quick-release pressure. Use two forks to shred the meat.

8. For the cauliflower rice: Break cauliflower into florets; chop the onion and mince the garlic. Use a food processor to pulse the cauliflower florets into a rice-like texture.

9. Heat the coconut oil in a skillet over medium heat. Sauté the onion and garlic for 3–4 minutes, or until the onion is translucent.

10. Add in the cauliflower rice and sauté for an additional 4–5 minutes. Season with salt.

11. Serve the beef on top of bowls of cauliflower rice with avocado, carrots, spinach, green onions, and remaining cilantro.

Beef Bone Broth:

Adapted from Nourishing Traditions

Ingredients:

4 pounds beef marrow and knuckle bones
1 calf's foot (or 3 chicken feet), cut into pieces
1/2 cup vinegar
4 or more quarts, cold filtered water
3 pounds meaty rib or neck bones
3 onions, coarsely chopped
3 carrots, coarsely chopped
3 celery stalks, coarsely chopped
Several sprigs of fresh thyme, tied together
1 teaspoon dried green peppercorns, crushed
1 bunch parsley

Directions:

1. Preheat the oven to 350 degrees.
2. Place the knuckle and marrow bones and calf's foot in a very large pot with vinegar and cover with water. Let stand for one hour.
3. Meanwhile, place the meaty bones in a roasting pan and brown in the oven. When well browned, add to the pot, along with the onions, carrots, and celery.
4. Pour the fat out of the roasting pan, add some cold water to the pan, set over a high flame, and bring to a boil, stirring with a wooden spoon to loosen up coagulated juices. Add this liquid to the pot you have filled with 4 or more quarts of cold, filtered water. Add additional water, if necessary, to cover the bones, but the liquid should come no higher than within one

inch of the rim of the pot, as the volume expands slightly during cooking.

5. Bring the pot to a boil. A large amount of scum will come to the top, and it is important to remove it with a spoon. After you have skimmed the scum, reduce the heat and add the thyme and peppercorns.

6. Simmer the stock for 12 hours. The longer you cook the stock, the richer and more flavorful it will be. However, the longer cooked stock also contains higher levels of histamines, which can be very inflammatory. So keep your cook time to 12 hours or under until the inflammation in your body is very low (you will be able to tell that inflammation is low when your red flag symptoms subside).

7. About 10 minutes before finishing the stock, add parsley. This will impart additional mineral ions to the broth. You will now have a pot of rather repulsive-looking brown liquid containing globs of gelatinous and fatty material. It won't even smell particularly good. But don't fret—after straining you will have a delicious and nourishing clear broth that is the ultimate tonic for lasting and thriving health.

8. Let soup cool down to slightly warmer than room temperature. Remove bones with tongs or a slotted spoon.

9. Strain the stock into a large bowl. Reserve in the refrigerator and remove the congealed fat that rises to the top. Break the soup up into batches (I use 12-ounce mason jars) and freeze most of the broth immediately, leaving in the fridge only what you will consume over the next 2 to 3 days.

Beef Stroganoff (in slow cooker):

Makes 8 Servings

Ingredients:

2 lbs beef stew meat

2 tsp sea salt

1 can full-fat coconut milk (plus a little more for deglazing the pan)

A package of mushrooms

3 carrots, sliced

1 cup bone broth

2 cloves garlic, minced

2 tbsp coconut oil

2 scoops Vital Proteins Beef Gelatin

Directions:

1. Turn on the slow cooker and set to low.
2. Over med-high heat melt coconut oil in a skillet.
3. Add cubed stew meat in batches to sear, then move the meat to the slow cooker.
4. In the same pan (add a little more coconut oil if it's all gone) saute mushrooms and garlic until mushrooms are browned.
5. Add a little coconut milk to the pan and scrape any meat and garlic goodness from the bottom of the pan and stir. Pour mushroom mixture into a slow cooker.
6. When the liquid comes to a boil, scoop out about a cup, mix in beef gelatin and stir until completely dissolved, pour the liquid back into the slow cooker.
7. Add remaining ingredients and cook on low for 7 hours.

Beets and Berries Smoothie:

Makes 1 Serving

Ingredients:

2 cups packed baby spinach (or leafy green of choice), blanched
1 cup berries of your choice
1/2 cup peeled and chopped beets, cooked
1/2 cup coconut milk
1/2 cup water
2 scoops collagen peptides
juice of 1/2 lemon

Directions:

1. Blend all ingredients until smooth

Beth's Berry Brothie:

Makes 1 Serving

Ingredients:

8 oz. bone broth of your choice (chicken is mildest)

Handful of blueberries

4 strawberries

A handful of spinach, blanched (or 2 scoops Amazing Grass greens powder)

1 tbsp coconut butter

2 scoops Vital Proteins Collagen Peptides

1 tbsp beet powder (I like Love Beets brand, you could also use blanched fresh beets)

Directions:

1. Blend! And drink that bad boy down!

Bone Broth Egg Drop Soup:

Ingredients:

2 cups bone broth

1 egg yolk

1/4 teaspoon ginger, minced

1 tablespoon spinach, coarsely chopped

1 tablespoon scallions, finely chopped

1/4 teaspoon salt

Directions:

1. Heat bone broth until rapidly boiling.
2. While the broth boils, whisk one whole egg (if you're eating the white as well; if you're just eating the yolk then only whisk the yolk) in a small bowl.
3. Drizzle egg slowly into the boiling broth, while mixing in with a fork. The egg should cook immediately.
4. Add ginger, spinach, scallions, and salt and simmer for another 1 to 3 minutes until the scallions are soft. Serve warm!

Note: Some mornings, when I'm in a rush, I just add a whisked egg yolk, handful of spinach, and few dashes of sea salt to boiling bone broth, and it's delicious.

Breakfast Casserole:

Ingredients:

1/2 spaghetti squash
1 1/2 carrots
1/2 onion
1 stalk celery
1/2 bunch kale
1/2 pound ground pork
1 1/2 teaspoons coconut oil
7 ounces coconut milk
1 1/2 teaspoons oregano
1/2 teaspoon garlic powder
1/2 teaspoon sea salt, to taste

Directions:

1. Preheat the oven to 375F.
2. In a shallow, non-reactive baking dish, roast squash for 30-45 minutes, or until squash can be punctured with a fork. When cool enough to handle, slice in half and scrape out the squash strands. Squash can be cooked ahead of time and refrigerated until ready to use.
3. Meanwhile, chop carrots, onion, celery, and kale.
4. In a skillet, brown ground pork and set aside.
5. In a separate pan, melt coconut oil. Add onions, carrots, and celery and saute for 7-10 minutes.
6. Add ground pork back to the pan. Stir in coconut milk, oregano, garlic powder, and salt. Simmer for 6-8 minutes.
7. Place spaghetti squash strands in a baking dish. Pour meat sauce over the squash, add chopped kale, and stir to combine. Bake for 40-45 minutes.
8. Remove from the oven and let the casserole sit for 5-10 minutes before serving.

Breakfast Hash:

Adapted from Real Plans
Makes 4 Servings

Ingredients:

1 large sweet potato
2 cloves garlic
1 onion
1/4 teaspoon fresh ginger
1 1/2 teaspoons extra virgin olive oil
1/2 pound ground pork
1 1/2 teaspoons maple syrup, optional
1/2 teaspoon dried sage
1/2 teaspoon dried rosemary
1/8 teaspoon cinnamon
1 teaspoon coarse sea salt, plus more to taste
8 ounces spinach

Directions:

1. Peel and chop sweet potato. Crush garlic. Peel and chop the onion. Grate ginger.
2. In a skillet, sauté oil and garlic over medium heat for 1 minute.
3. Add in chopped sweet potato and stir.
4. After 4-5 minutes, add in the onion.
5. Let sauté for about 5 minutes, stirring occasionally.
6. Mix in ground pork, syrup, sage, rosemary, cinnamon, ginger, and salt. Break sausage into small pieces as you stir. Cook until the sausage is no longer pink.
7. Mix in fresh spinach, and cook for 2-3 minutes, or until sautéed.
8. Remove skillet from heat and serve hot.

Broccoli Salad with Cranberries:

Adapted from Real Plans
Makes 4 Servings

Ingredients:

4 heads broccoli

1/2 cup frozen cranberries (thawed)

2 tablespoons coconut aminos

1 tablespoon honey

1/2 lemon

2 teaspoons coarse sea salt

1/2 teaspoon garlic powder

1/2 teaspoon ground ginger

1/4 cup extra virgin olive oil

Directions:

1. Chop broccoli and cranberries and blanch. (Or saute in coconut oil, whatever you prefer)
2. Juice the lemon.
3. Mix everything together and let sit for about 30 min so the flavors come together.

Cauliflower Rice:

Adapted from Real Plans
Makes 2 Servings

Ingredients:

1/2 onion
1 teaspoon minced garlic
1/2 head cauliflower
1 tablespoon extra virgin olive oil, or fat of choice
coarse sea salt, to taste

Directions:

1. Chop onion. Break cauliflower into florets, then use a food processor to pulse the cauliflower florets into a rice-like texture.
2. Heat oil in a skillet over medium heat.
3. Sauté the onion and garlic for 3–4 minutes, or until the onion is translucent.
4. Add in the cauliflower rice and sauté for an additional 4–5 minutes.
5. Season with salt.

Chicken and Asparagus Stir Fry:

Adapted from Real Plans
Makes 4 Servings

Ingredients:

2/3 lemon
2/3 cup bone broth
4 teaspoons fish sauce
2 green onions
1/3 inch fresh ginger
2 cloves garlic
1 pound asparagus
2 tablespoons fresh mint
2 tablespoons coconut oil
2 cups cooked chicken
2 teaspoons arrowroot
4 teaspoons filtered water
coarse sea salt, to taste

Directions:

1. Zest and juice the lemon.
2. In a small bowl, combine the stock, fish sauce, sucanat, lemon zest, and lemon juice for the sauce.
3. Chop the green onions, keeping the green and white parts separate. Peel and grate the ginger and mince the garlic. Remove the woody ends from the asparagus and slice them lengthwise and cut into thirds. Chop the mint.
4. In a wok or large frying pan heat coconut oil over medium-high heat.
5. Add the ginger, garlic, and whites of onions. Sauté for 15-20 seconds to release the flavors.

6. Add sauce and the asparagus; cover, cooking for 2-3 minutes - until the asparagus turns bright green.

7. Toss in the shredded chicken and heat through.

8. Mix the arrowroot with the filtered water and add this mixture to the pan, cooking until the sauce begins to thicken (2-3 minutes).

9. Toss in the mint and green bits of onion. Adjust seasoning with sea salt. Serve.

Chicken Bone Broth:

Adapted from Nourishing Traditions

Ingredients:

4 quarts cold filtered water

2 tablespoons vinegar

1 large onion, coarsely chopped

2 carrots, peeled and coarsely chopped

3 celery stalks, coarsely chopped

1 whole free-range chicken or 2 to 3 pounds of bony chicken parts, such as necks, backs, breastbones, and wings*

Gizzards from one chicken (optional)

2 to 4 chicken feet

1 bunch parsley

Note: Farm-raised, free-range chickens give the best results. Conventionally-raised chickens will not produce stock that gels

Directions:

1. Fill a stockpot with water, vinegar, onion, carrots, and celery. If you are using a whole chicken, put the whole chicken (removing the gizzard bag) in the stockpot; if you're using chicken pieces, put all of them in the stockpot. Add in gizzards and chicken feet. Let stand 60 minutes (this process helps break the bones down, don't skip!)

2. Bring the pot to a boil, and remove scum that rises to the top. Reduce heat, cover, and simmer for 8 to 12 hours. The longer you cook the stock, the richer and more flavorful it will be. However, the longer cooked stock also contains higher levels of histamines, which can be very inflammatory. So keep your cook time to 12 hours or under until the inflammation in your

body is very low (you will be able to tell that inflammation is low when your red flag symptoms subside).

3. About 10 minutes before finishing the stock, add parsley. This will impart additional mineral ions to the broth.

4. Let soup cool down a bit until it's a little warmer than room temperature (or basically not too hot for you to get the chicken pieces out). Remove whole chicken or pieces with a slotted spoon or strain the broth. You can reserve the chicken meat for other uses, such as chicken salads, enchiladas, sandwiches, or curries.

5. Strain the stock into a large bowl and reserve it in your refrigerator and remove the congealed fat that rises to the top. Break the soup up into batches (I use 12-ounce mason jars) and freeze most of the broth immediately, leaving in the fridge only what you will consume over the next 2 to 3 days.

Chicken Broccoli and Sweet Potato Sheet Pan Dinner:

Adapted from 30 Min AIP
Makes 2 Servings

Ingredients:

1 lb sweet potatoes
Avocado oil
½ tsp salt
½ lb broccoli
1 lb boneless, skinless chicken thighs
½ tsp garlic powder
½ tsp onion powder
1 tsp oregano
1 tsp parsley

Directions:

1. Place large baking sheet in the oven and set the oven to 425° F.
2. Peel sweet potatoes and dice into ½-inch cubes. Toss with 1 tbsp avocado oil and salt.
3. Remove pan from oven and spread sweet potatoes on baking sheet. Put the baking sheet back in the oven. Wash and cut up broccoli into spears.
4. Pat chicken dry, and cut into 1-inch pieces.
5. Remove sheet pan from oven. Toss the sweet potatoes and add broccoli, chicken, and 1 tablespoon avocado oil to the baking sheet.
6. Cook in the oven for an additional 12 minutes.

Chicken Marbella:

Adapted from Real Plans
makes 2 servings

Ingredients:

1 1/2 cloves garlic

1 pound boneless, skinless chicken thighs

1 tablespoon extra virgin olive oil

3 tablespoons apple cider vinegar

1 1/2 ounces capers

3 ounces green olives, pitted

1 1/2 teaspoons oregano

1 bay leaf

1/2 teaspoon sea salt, to taste

Directions:

1. Preheat the oven to 350F.
2. Peel and finely chop garlic.
3. Combine all ingredients in an oven-safe baking dish. Season with sea salt. Flip the chicken pieces over a few times to make sure they are coated in the mixture.
4. Bake for 25 minutes or until done, remove from the oven, and serve.

Chinese Soup with Roasted Veggies:

Adapted from Real Plans
Makes 2 Servings

Ingredients:

1/2 small butternut squash
1/2 onion
2 1/2 carrots
2 stalks celery
1/2 teaspoon coarse sea salt, plus more to taste
1/2 head garlic
1 cup cooked chicken
2 cups chicken bone broth
1/2 bunch kale
1/2 cup fresh herbs, (chives basil cilantro parsley or anything you have on hand)

Directions:

1. Peel and deseed squash. Chop onion, carrots, celery, and squash into bite-sized chunks, season with sea salt, and place on a lipped baking sheet lined with silpat or parchment. Roast with the whole head of garlic at 350F for about 1 hour, or until the vegetables start to soften. Set aside.
2. Shred the chicken and add with chicken broth into a stockpot. Mash the roasted garlic and mix with some of the chicken broth to make a thin paste.
3. Add the garlic paste and roasted veggies into the soup; cook on low for 30 minutes to 1 hour.
4. Mince the kale and herbs finely and add to the soup; allow them to brighten for a minute or two. Season with additional sea salt and freshly ground pepper, ladle into bowls and serve.

Chinese Shredded Beef with Broccoli:

Adapted from Real Plans
Makes 4 Servings

Ingredients:

1 orange
2/3 cup beef bone broth (or bone broth of choice)
4 teaspoons fish sauce
2 green onions
1/3 inch fresh ginger
2 cloves garlic
1 small head of broccoli
2 tablespoons coconut oil
2 cups shredded beef
2 teaspoons arrowroot
4 teaspoons filtered water
coarse sea salt, to taste

Directions:

1. Zest and juice the orange.
2. In a small bowl, combine the stock, fish sauce, orange zest, and orange juice for the sauce.
3. Chop the green onions, keeping the green and white parts separate. Peel and grate the ginger and mince the garlic. Separate broccoli into florets.
4. In a wok or large frying pan heat coconut oil over medium-high heat.
5. Add the ginger, garlic, and whites of onions. Sauté for 15-20 seconds to release the flavors.
6. Add sauce and the broccoli; cover, cooking for 2-3 minutes - until the broccoli turns bright green.

7. Toss in the shredded beef and heat through.
8. Mix the arrowroot with the filtered water and add this mixture to the pan, cooking until the sauce begins to thicken (2-3 minutes).
9. Toss in the green bits of onion. Adjust seasoning with sea salt. Serve.

Coconut Baked Shrimp:

Adapted from Real Plans
makes 2 servings

Ingredients:

3/4 pound wild-caught shrimp

3 cloves garlic

1 1/2 tablespoons flat-leaf parsley

1/4 cup coconut oil

2 1/2 tablespoons bone broth

2 teaspoons coarse sea salt

1/3 cup coconut flakes

1/4 small lemon

Directions:

1. Preheat oven to 425F.
2. Devein and peel the shrimp. Mince the garlic and parsley, and melt the oil.
3. In a bowl, combine the shrimp, garlic, and broth.
4. Place shrimp mixture in a shallow baking dish in a single layer.
5. Season with salt.
6. Using the same bowl mix melted oil, coconut flakes, and parsley until well combined.
7. Using your fingers, sprinkle the mixture evenly over the shrimp.
8. Bake about 15 minutes or until the shrimp are pink and opaque and the topping is nicely browned.
9. Serve with a squeeze of lemon.

Coconut Cauliflower Rice:

Adapted from Real Plans
Makes 4 servings

Ingredients:

1 head cauliflower
1 lime
2 tablespoons cilantro
8 ounces coconut milk
coarse sea salt, to taste

Directions:

1. Coarsely chop the cauliflower. Juice the lime and chop cilantro.
2. Place the chopped cauliflower in a food processor and pulse until it reaches a rice-like texture.
3. Add the cauliflower, coconut milk, and optional honey to a saucepan. Bring to a boil. Let simmer for around 8-10 minutes until cauliflower softens and is cooked to your liking. It will be somewhat creamy. For a less creamy texture, use a little less coconut milk.
4. Stir in the lime juice and cilantro. Season with sea salt to your preference and enjoy.

Coconut Porridge:

From Real Plans
makes 2 servings

Ingredients:

1 cup coconut milk
1/4 cup filtered water
6 tablespoons coconut flour
4 tablespoons shredded coconut
1 banana
berries

Directions:

1. In a small saucepan, mix together the liquid, coconut flour, and shredded coconut. Bring to a boil (mixture will be thick), cover, reduce heat to low, and simmer for 2-3 minutes. Stir halfway through.
2. Mash banana, then whisk into the mixture and serve immediately, topped with fresh berries.

Coconut Turmeric Bites (Fat Bombs):

Ingredients:

1 cup coconut butter (also called coconut cream concentrate or coconut mana)

3/4 cup shredded coconut + 1/2 tsp for topping (I highly recommend tropical traditions for this)

1 tbsp coconut milk (or water)

1 tsp coconut oil

2 tsp turmeric

1/2 tsp cinnamon

Directions:

1. Add the coconut butter and the shredded coconut to a mixing bowl and stir well to combine. You want the coconut butter to be **softened** (but **not melted**), so depending on the consistency of yours, heat it in a double boiler over the stove if needed.
2. Add the remaining ingredients and combine.
3. Begin rolling the dough into balls about 1" – 1 ¼" in diameter, (or you can easily choose whichever size you'd like) and place onto a plate lined with parchment paper.
4. If desired, sprinkle about 1/2 tsp of shredded coconut on top of the bites.
5. Put the turmeric bites into the refrigerator and chill for a minimum of 30 minutes, or in the freezer for more of a bite.
6. Remove from the fridge and enjoy! Note that these are best enjoyed cold.

Deconstructed Egg Rolls:

Adapted from Real Plans
Makes 4 servings

Ingredients:

1 head green cabbage
3 carrots
1 onion
5 cloves garlic
1-inch fresh ginger
4 green onions
1 tablespoon coconut oil
1 pound ground pork
1/2 cup coconut aminos
coarse sea salt, to taste

Directions:

1. Shred cabbage and carrot. Dice onion. Mince garlic. Grate ginger. Slice green onions.
2. Heat coconut oil in a skillet. Add onion and cook until it begins to soften. Add pork and break it apart with a wooden spoon, cooking until it is no longer pink.
3. Meanwhile, in a small bowl combine garlic, coconut aminos, and ginger; set aside.
4. Once ground pork is cooked through, add cabbage and carrots to the skillet and stir to combine.
5. Pour sauce mixture into the skillet and stir, continuing to cook over medium heat for about 5-15 minutes or until cabbage is wilted.
6. Season with salt, to taste. Top with sliced green onion and serve.

Fish Bone Broth:

Adapted from Nourishing Traditions

Ideally, fish stock is made from the bones of the sole or turbot. In Europe, you can buy these fish on the bone. The fishmonger skins and filets the fish for you, giving you the filets for your evening meal and the bones for making the stock and final sauce. Unfortunately, in America sole arrives at the fish market preboned. But snapper, rockfish, and other non-oily fish work equally well, and a good fish merchant will save the carcasses for you if you ask them. As they normally throw these carcasses away, they shouldn't charge you for them. Be sure to take the heads as well as the body — these are especially rich in iodine and fat-soluble vitamins. Classic cooking texts advise against using oily fish such as salmon for making broth, probably because highly unsaturated fish oils become rancid during the long cooking process.

Ingredients:

2 tablespoons cultured ghee
2 onions, coarsely chopped
1 carrot, coarsely chopped
1/2 cup dry white wine or vermouth
3 or 4 whole carcasses, including heads, of non-oily fish such as sole, turbot, rockfish, or snapper
1/4 cup vinegar
About 3 quarts cold filtered water
Several sprigs of fresh thyme
Several sprigs of fresh parsley
1 bay leaf

Directions:

1. Melt ghee in a large stainless steel pot. Add the onions and carrot, and cook, until they are soft (about a half-hour).
2. Add wine and bring to a boil.
3. Add the fish carcasses and cover them with cold, filtered water. Add vinegar. Bring to a boil and skim off the scum and impurities as they rise to the top.
4. Add the thyme and parsley to the pot (you can tie them with twine or keep them loose). Reduce heat, cover, and simmer for 8 to 12 hours.
5. Remove carcasses with tongs or a slotted spoon, and strain the liquid into pint-sized storage containers. Reserve in the refrigerator and remove the congealed fat that rises to the top. Break the soup up into batches (I use 12-ounce mason jars) and freeze most of the broth immediately, leaving in the fridge only what you will consume over the next 2 to 3 days.

Fruit Bowl with Coconut Butter:

Adapted from Real Plans
Makes 1 Serving

Ingredients:

1 nectarine, or peaches
1/8 cup blueberries
1/8 cup raspberries
1 1/2 tablespoons coconut butter
sea salt

Directions:

1. Melt coconut butter in a double boiler.
2. Chop fruit into bite-sized pieces, drizzle with melted coconut butter, and sprinkle with a pinch of sea salt.

Garden Green Brothie:

Adapted from Brodo (shared on Instagram)
Makes 1 Serving

Ingredients:

1 cup kale
1 cup spinach
½ green apple
2 tbsp parsley
½ mango
½ banana
Juice of half a lemon
2 tsp coconut oil
8 oz chicken bone broth (or bone broth of your choice)

Directions:

1. Blend, baby blend!

Ginger Lime Salmon Bowls:

Adapted from Real Plans
Makes 2 Servings

Ingredients:

For the noodles:
1 zucchini
1 carrot
coarse sea salt
For the salmon:
2 limes
2/3 inch fresh ginger
1 tablespoon coconut vinegar
1/4 teaspoon garlic powder
3/4 pound salmon, 6-ounce filet per person
1/2 bunch kale
1 1/2 green onions
1/2 avocado
extra virgin olive oil, for kale
coarse sea salt, to taste
For the dressing:
1 1/2 teaspoons coconut vinegar
1 1/2 teaspoons avocado oil
1 teaspoon honey

Directions:

1. For the noodles:
2. To make zucchini and carrot noodles, either purchase: a julienne peeler or a spiral cutter OR simply use a sharp knife to cut the zucchini and carrot first lengthwise into strips, then

slice those strips as finely as possible into spaghetti-like pieces.

3. Sprinkle some sea salt over the noodles and let them sit for 25 minutes in the sink to sweat out excess water. After 25 minutes, rinse well to remove excess salt and pat dry with a paper towel.

4. Cook in a large pan over medium heat for about 2 minutes, to allow the noodles to soften slightly. Remove from heat.

5. For the salmon:

6. Juice half of the limes for the marinade. Quarter lime (one slice per serving for garnish). Peel and grate the ginger.

7. In a shallow dish big enough to hold the salmon in a single layer, combine ginger, coconut vinegar, lime juice, and garlic powder. Add the salmon filets and refrigerate for 2-3 hours.

8. Preheat oven to 425F.

9. Remove the tough center stalk from kale and toss in a little olive oil and sea salt. Set aside. prepare garnishes: Slice green onions thinly on the diagonal; peel and thinly slice avocado.

10. Remove the salmon from the marinade and place on a baking sheet lined with parchment paper or silpat. Bake for about 15 minutes until the salmon is nearly cooked through.

11. Switch the oven to the high broiling setting. Add the kale in a single layer to the same baking sheet as the fish. Cook 1-2 minutes with the oven ajar until the kale has crisped. Watch closely to avoid burning the kale. Remove from oven.

12. Juice remaining lime for dressing. In a small bowl whisk together all of the dressing ingredients, including the lime juice.

13. To each serving bowl add zucchini and carrot noodles, salmon, and kale. Garnish with sliced avocado, green onions, and a lime wedge. Drizzle with dressing and serve.

Golden Milk Bone Broth:

Ingredients:

4 cups bone broth

1 cup whole fat coconut milk

1 teaspoon ground turmeric

1 teaspoon ground ginger

2 to 4 cloves of garlic, smashed and peeled

Pepper, freshly ground

Sea salt

Directions:

1. Combine all ingredients into a saucepan and heat.

Ham and White Sweet Potato Hash:

Adapted from Real Plans
makes 4 servings

Ingredients:

3 white sweet potatoes
4 tablespoons coconut oil
1 teaspoon garlic powder
1 teaspoon oregano
1 teaspoon dried rosemary
1 teaspoon coarse sea salt, plus more to taste
2 cups ham
8 ounces spinach

Directions:

1. Preheat the oven to 400F and line a baking tray.
2. Peel and cube the sweet potatoes. Warm the coconut oil so that it is liquid, if necessary.
3. In a large bowl, toss the sweet potato cubes with seasonings and half of the coconut oil. Add salt to taste.
4. Spread the cubes out on the lined baking tray in a single layer: bake for 20 - 25 minutes, or until a fork can pierce a potato cube easily but firmly.
5. Remove the tray of potatoes from the oven and set it aside on a cooling rack.
6. In a large skillet, heat the remaining coconut oil over medium heat.
7. Fry potatoes in a single layer (do multiple batches if necessary) for 5-8 minutes, tossing every minute or so to brown on all sides, and be done to your desired level of crispiness.

8. Cube the cooked ham if not already in bite-sized pieces.
9. At the end, toss in the cooked ham and cook until warm through. Add the spinach and cook until it is just wilted. Serve immediately.

Happy Egg Mayo:

Ingredients:

2 egg yolks
3 tsp lemon juice, divided
½ cup extra virgin olive oil
½ cup coconut oil, melted
Sea salt & pepper to taste

Directions:

1. In a blender or food processor mix yolks and 1 tsp lemon juice.
2. In a separate bowl whisk together olive and coconut oils.
3. Set blender to low and SLOWLY pour in the oil mixture (even a drop at a time in the beginning). You're creating an emulsion so if you put in too much oil at once the mayo will "break" and will be difficult to save.
4. As you add more oil the mayo will start to thicken up and you can begin to pour the oil faster.
5. Once all the oil is incorporated and your mayo is nice and thick- whisk in the rest of the lemon juice.
6. Stir in salt & pepper to taste.

Hollandaise Sauce:

Ingredients:

½ cup melted ghee
2 egg yolks
1 Tablespoon lemon juice
Pinch of salt

Directions:

1. Gently melt the ghee on the stovetop. It shouldn't be boiling hot.
2. Place the egg yolks, lemon juice, and salt in the blender.
3. Start the blender on low and run for about 30 seconds then SLOWLY drizzle the melted ghee into the blender through the hole in the lid. You must go slow or the emulsion will separate and get soupy.
4. Once all the ghee is added and the Hollandaise has thickened, you're done. Scrape it out and use on eggs, roasted veggies, a juicy steak, whatever your heart desires.

Key Lime Pie Fat Bombs:

Ingredients:

2 cup coconut oil, melted

1 cup coconut butter

3/4 cup key lime juice

Directions:

1. Put all ingredients in a food processor and blend until well combined.
2. Spread into a 9x9 (or similar) pan and place in freezer. (Optional: line pan with parchment paper for easier removal)
3. Remove from freezer once solid and cut into 1" x 1" cubes. Store in fridge or freezer.

Optional: If you'd like fun shapes use silicone candy molds rather than a square or rectangular pan.

Lemony Fat Bombs:

Ingredients:

2 cup coconut oil, melted
1 cup coconut butter
1-2 tbsp lemon zest

Directions:

1. Put all ingredients in a food processor and blend until well combined.
2. Spread into a 9x9 (or similar) pan and place in freezer. (Optional: line pan with parchment paper for easier removal)
3. Remove from freezer once solid and cut into 1"x 1" cubes. Store in fridge or freezer.

Optional: If you'd like fun shapes use silicone candy molds rather than a square or rectangular pan.

Liver Support Soup:

Ingredients:

4 beets, cooked

3 carrots, blanched

1-inch piece fresh ginger, peeled and minced

4 to 6 pieces of fresh turmeric (or 1 heaping tsp ground turmeric)

1 large handful of cilantro, stems included

1 large handful of dandelion greens, stems included, blanched

1 large handful of parsley

Juice of 2 lemons

1/4 teaspoon freshly ground black pepper

1/4 teaspoon sea salt

1 garlic clove (or 1/4 tsp organic garlic powder for a milder flavor)

3 cup of bone broth

1/2 cup of filtered water

Directions:

1. Blend all ingredients until smooth.
2. Separate into 8 oz servings
3. Heat one serving in a saucepan and serve

Alternate: in Phase 3- instead of heating add some blueberries and blend with one serving and drink as a smoothie.

Mango Mint Green Smoothie:

Adapted from Whole Foods
Serves 2

Ingredients:

2 cups baby spinach or roughly chopped spinach leaves (about 2 ounces)
1 can full-fat coconut milk
1/2 cup lightly packed fresh mint leaves
1/4 cup lime juice
1 large or 2 small ripe, juicy mangoes, roughly chopped
1 small banana (optional)

Directions:

1. In a blender, purée spinach, coconut milk, mint, lime juice, and mangoes until smooth. Taste and add a banana for extra sweetness, if desired. Serve immediately.

Mangu:

Adapted from Real Plans
Makes 2 Servings

Ingredients:

2 green plantains
sea salt, to taste
1 cup water, plus more for boiling
1/2 yellow onion
1 1/2 teaspoons extra virgin olive oil
1 teaspoon apple cider vinegar
1/2 avocado

Directions:

1. Cut ends off plantains and make two shallow lengthwise. Cut plantains into thirds horizontally and slice the thirds in half lengthwise.
2. Place plantains in a pot and cover with water. Lightly salt. Bring water to a boil and allow plantains to cook until tender.
3. In the meantime, thinly slice onion and slice avocados.
4. Heat olive oil in a pan over medium heat. Add onions and cook until translucent.
5. Add vinegar and season with salt to taste. Remove from heat.
6. When the plantains are tender, remove from heat and drain, reserving a cup of cooking water.
7. Mash plantains with a potato masher adding cool filtered water until it reaches a creamy consistency, you might not use all of the cool water. You can also use an immersion blender. Plantains absorb a lot of water so make sure you add enough to prevent it from drying and hardening. Once creamy, add some of the warm reserved water to the prepared plantains.
8. Divide mangu (mashed plantains) among plates, top with sauteed onions, and place sliced avocados on the side.

Maple Chicken Breakfast Sausage:

Adapted from Real Plans
Makes 4 Servings

Ingredients:

1 pound ground chicken
2 tablespoons maple syrup
2 teaspoons coarse sea salt
1 teaspoon dried sage
1 teaspoon dried parsley
1/2 teaspoon garlic powder
1/2 teaspoon onion powder
1/2 teaspoon dried thyme
1/4 teaspoon ground cinnamon
1/4 teaspoon ground cloves
1 tablespoon coconut oil, or bacon fat

Directions:

1. In a large mixing bowl, combine ground chicken, maple syrup, salt, sage, parsley, garlic powder, onion powder, thyme, cinnamon, and cloves.
2. Mix until all ingredients are well-incorporated.
3. Form into patties.
4. Melt coconut oil or bacon fat in a skillet over medium heat until shimmering.
5. In small batches, cook until browned on both sides and cooked all the way through. Serve.

Mixed Veggie Noodles with Pork:

Adapted from Real Plans
Makes 4 Servings

Ingredients:

3 carrots

4 scallions

2 limes

2 zucchinis

2 summer squash

2 tablespoons coconut aminos, plus more to taste

2 tablespoons extra virgin olive oil

1/2 teaspoon garlic powder

1/2 teaspoon onion powder

2 cups shredded pork

4 nori sheets, optional

Directions:

1. Peel carrots. Mince scallions. Juice the limes.
2. Either by hand or with a julienne tool, make veggie noodles from the carrots, zucchini, and summer squash.
3. In a large bowl, whisk together coconut aminos, lime juice, olive oil, garlic powder, and onion powder. Add veggie "noodles," scallions, and shredded pork; toss well.
4. To toast nori sheets, preheat oven to 200F. On an ungreased baking sheet, arrange nori in a single layer. Bake for 2 minutes. Remove from baking sheet, crush sheets, and use as garnish.
5. Serve at room temperature.

Morning Smoothie:

Adapted from The Paleo Mom
Makes 1 Serving

Ingredients:

1/2 banana
1/4-½ avocado
1 cup coconut milk or filtered water
2 to 3 cups fresh leafy greens (spinach, kale, lettuce, baby collards, etc.)
2 scoops Vital Proteins Collagen Peptides

Directions:

1. Place all the ingredients in a blender and blend on high for 1 to 2 minutes, until smooth.

NoMato Sauce:

Adapted from Amanda Torres

(Note: this recipe yields about 8 1/2 cups of sauce, so make a batch and freeze some of it for any time you want a marinara-like sauce. It's great over zoodles!)

Ingredients:

2 to 4 tablespoons of grass-fed ghee or coconut oil
4 ribs celery, chopped
1 large onion, chopped
3 medium beets, chopped
1 pound carrots, chopped
Enough bone broth to barely cover all ingredients; (about 2 cups; use less for a thicker sauce)
4 to 8 cloves garlic, pressed or finely minced
1/2 teaspoon dried basil
1/2 teaspoon dried oregano
1/2 teaspoon dried thyme
1/4 teaspoon dried marjoram
2 dried bay leaves
Juice from 2 lemons
15 to 20 kalamata olives, pitted
Sea salt and pepper to taste

Directions:

1. Heat fat of choice in a large pot over medium-low heat for several minutes.
2. Add garlic, celery, and onion to pot and cook, stirring a few times, until onion is translucent.
3. Add beets and carrots and cook until soft stirring a few times.

4. Add broth, using just enough to cover the ingredients (or less for a thicker, less watery sauce).

5. Add dried herbs (basil, marjoram, oregano, bay leaves, and thyme) and lemon juice and stir well to combine everything. Bring to a boil, then reduce heat to a simmer and cover. Simmer for about 30 minutes, or until all vegetables are tender. Stir about halfway through cooking.

6. Cool sauce, remove bay leaves and blend in a blender. (Avoid putting a very hot sauce into a plastic blender as chemicals will leach out into your food.)

7. Add the kalamata olives and salt and pepper to taste.

One-Dish Roasted Brats with Apples and Butternut Squash:

Adapted from Whole Foods
Makes 8-10 servings

Ingredients:

1 medium butternut squash, peeled and cut into 1/2-inch cubes (about 2 1/2 cups)

2 apples, sliced

1 cup seedless red grapes

1 small red onion, halved and cut into thick slices

2 teaspoons coconut oil

1 teaspoon crushed caraway seeds

3/4 teaspoon fine sea salt

12 fresh bratwursts (or any AIP friendly mild sausage)

Directions:

1. Preheat the oven to 450°F. Put coconut oil in a large roasting pan or rimmed baking sheet and place in oven until oil is melted, then remove. Add squash, apples, grapes, and onion. Sprinkle with caraway seeds and salt and toss to coat. Arrange brats over the top. Roast until brats are browned and hot all the way through, and squash is very tender, about 35 minutes.

Pancit:

Adapted from Real Plans
Makes 4 Servings

Ingredients:

2 tablespoons coconut oil

3 cloves garlic

1 bunch green onion

4 carrots

1 head green cabbage

1/2 pound chicken breast, or boneless chicken thighs

1/2 pound shrimp

2 cups cooked pork

1 teaspoon coarse sea salt

3 tablespoons coconut aminos, plus more to taste

3 tablespoons fish sauce, plus more to taste

1/4 cup bone broth

1 lemon

Directions:

1. In a wok or large pan heat the coconut oil over medium-high heat.
2. Mince the garlic, dice the onions, grate carrots and slice the cabbage into ribbons.
3. Add the garlic, cabbage, whites of onions, and carrots and cook for about 10-15 minutes, until cabbage is tender.
4. Chop chicken into 1/2 inch cubes. Remove tail and shells and devein shrimp. Chop pork into ½ inch pieces.
5. Add the chicken and sauté with the raw shrimp and sea salt. Cook until shrimp are pink.

6. Add the pork, coconut aminos, fish sauce, onion greens, chicken broth. Cook just until heated through and well combined.

7. Finish with a squeeze of lemon to taste and extra fish sauce to taste.

Philly Steak Lettuce Cups:

From Real Plans
Makes 2 servings

Ingredients:

3/4 pound rib-eye steak
1 onion
1/4 pound cremini mushrooms
1 1/2 tablespoons bacon fat
coarse sea salt, to taste
1/2 head romaine lettuce

Directions:

1. If your steak is not frozen, freeze it overnight so you can slice it thinly. Remove from the freezer and using your sharpest knife, slice the steak as thinly as possible. Slice the onions.
2. In a skillet over medium-high heat, sauté the onions and mushrooms in bacon fat. Remove to a plate.
3. Turn heat to high. Add the rib eye steak and season generously with sea salt. Cook for a couple of minutes until browned.
4. Replace veggies into the pan with the meat and reduce heat to low. Cover and cook for about 2 minutes.
5. Wash and separate the leaves of lettuce and serve the veggie and meat mix in the lettuce leaves.

Plantain Pancakes:

Adapted from Real Plans
makes 2 servings (recipe only for Phase 1 Phase and Phase 4)

Ingredients:

1 1/2 green plantains

1/4 cup coconut oil, plus more for greasing pan

1 cup filtered water

1 teaspoon gelatin

1/2 teaspoon sea salt

1/4 cup arrowroot

Directions:

1. Peel and chop the plantains. Melt coconut oil.
2. Place all ingredients in a high speed blender or food processor
3. Turn on and push ingredients down with the tamper until it is uniform and smooth. If you need to add a bit more water, you can do so. You want the batter to be thick, but pourable.
4. Heat a large cast iron or nonstick pan with coconut oil.
5. Using a 1/4 measuring cup, cook pancakes in small batches, flipping when the batter begins to bubble. You'll need to cook for several minutes on each side.
6. Serve immediately.

Plantain Waffles

Adapted from Real Plans
makes 2 servings (recipe only for Phase 1 and Phase 4)

Ingredients:

1 1/2 green plantains
1/4 cup coconut oil, plus more for greasing waffle iron
1/2 cup filtered water
1 teaspoon Vital Proteins beef gelatin
1/2 teaspoon sea salt
1/4 cup arrowroot
maple syrup, to taste

Directions:

1. Peel and chop plantains. Melt coconut oil.
2. Place all ingredients in a high-speed blender or food processor.
3. Turn on and push ingredients down with the tamper until it is uniform and smooth. If you need to add a bit more water, you can do so. You want the batter to be thick, but pourable.
4. Heat your waffle iron, coat with coconut oil, and cook per instructions. I sometimes let it go a little longer than the regular waffles as it can take a little longer to brown.
5. Serve immediately drizzled with a touch of maple syrup.

Pork and Bok Choy Stir Fry

Adapted from Real Plans
Makes 4 servings

Ingredients:

1 small lemon
2/3 cup bone broth
4 teaspoons fish sauce
2 green onions
1 teaspoon fresh ginger
2 cloves garlic
1 bok choy
2 tablespoons coconut oil
2 cups shredded pork
coarse sea salt, to taste

Directions:

1. Zest and juice the lemon.
2. In a small bowl, combine the stock, fish sauce, lemon zest, and lemon juice for the sauce.
3. Chop the green onions, keeping the green and white parts separate. Peel and grate the ginger and mince the garlic. Trim and discard the thick base of the bok choy. Cut the stalk in half lengthwise. Slice the bok choy into bite-sized pieces.
4. In a wok or large frying pan heat coconut oil over medium-high heat.
5. Add the ginger, garlic, and whites of onions. Sauté for 15-20 seconds to release the flavors.
6. Add sauce and the bok choy; cover, cooking for 2-3 minutes - until the bok choy turns bright green.
7. Toss in the shredded pork and heat through.
8. Toss in the green bits of onion. Adjust seasoning with sea salt. Serve.

Phase 2 Smoothie

Ingredients:

1 cup of coconut yogurt or 1 cup of coconut milk (depending on your preferred thickness

1 cup of filtered water

½ avocado

1 scoop of Bone Broth Protein (I like the Ancient Nutrition brand)

1 scoop of Collagen Peptides (I like the Vital Proteins brand)

¼ teaspoon of cinnamon

1 teaspoon of turmeric

1 teaspoon of ground ginger

2 cups of blanched spinach or kale

¼ teaspoon of ground Himalayan sea salt

Directions:

1. Blend all ingredients; add 1/2 cup filtered water if too thick for your liking. Enjoy!

Note: Throw in some blueberries too as long as you're not in Phase 2

Radish Salad

Adapted from Real Plans
Makes 4 Servings

Ingredients:

1 bunch radish
1/2 lemon
coarse sea salt, to taste

Directions:

1. Using a food processor, slice the radishes as thinly as possible.
2. Juice the lemon.
3. Garnish with lemon juice and sea salt.

Red Beet & Apple Salad

Ingredients:

1 bunch fresh spinach, washed

2 red apples, quartered, cored, and thinly sliced

3 fresh beetroot, thinly sliced

Juice of 1 lemon

4 tablespoons olive oil

¼ teaspoon salt

1 tablespoon fresh oregano, finely chopped

Directions:

1. In a large bowl, toss together spinach, sliced apples, and sliced beets.
2. In a separate, smaller bowl, combine lemon juice, olive oil, and salt. Mix together with a whisk until the mixture is fully emulsified.
3. Toss the dressing and the salad, and then divide the salad onto serving plates.
4. Top each portion with fresh oregano, then serve.

Roasted Beets

Adapted from Real Plans
Makes 4 Servings

Ingredients:

1 pound beet
3 tablespoons coconut oil
1 teaspoon coarse sea salt

Directions:

1. Preheat oven to 375F.
2. Scrub and trim beets. Chop into one-inch chunks by first halving and quartering. No need to peel yet.
3. Place in a baking dish in a single layer, toss without about half of the olive oil, and roast in the oven until cooked through, approximately 45 to 60 minutes, or until beets are tender when pierced with a fork.
4. Remove from the oven, let cool for 10 minutes. The peels should slip off fairly easily with your hands. Use a sharp knife or vegetable peeler if you need extra help. Do this in the sink to minimize mess.
5. Place peeled beets back in a baking dish or a serving bowl. Toss with remaining olive oil and sea salt and serve.

Roasted Root Veggies

Adapted from Real Plans
Makes 4 Servings

Ingredients:

3 carrots

2 parsnips

1 sweet potato

2 tablespoons coconut oil, or fat of choice

1 teaspoon coarse sea salt, plus more to taste

Directions:

1. Preheat the oven to 450F.
2. Wash the carrots and parsnips, cut ends off, and chop into 1-inch pieces. Wash and chop the sweet potato.
3. Place the vegetables in a shallow baking dish just big enough to fit in a single layer along with your fat of choice.
4. Place dish, uncovered, on the center rack of the oven. After 20 minutes, gently turn the vegetables, coating well with the now-melted fat.
5. Season generously with sea salt and bake for about 30-40 minutes, until tender and lightly golden-brown.

Sausage and Butternut Squash Breakfast Skillet

Adapted from Real Plans
Makes 4 Servings

Ingredients:

1 1/2 onions
1 tablespoon minced garlic
1 small butternut squash
3 tablespoons extra virgin olive oil
1 1/2 pounds ground pork
1 teaspoon dried sage
1 teaspoon dried rosemary
1/2 teaspoon onion powder
2 teaspoons coarse sea salt
1/4 teaspoon cinnamon

Directions:

1. Dice onion. Peel, de-seed, and dice squash into small 1/2 inch cubes.
2. Heat oil in a saute pan over medium heat.
3. Add onion and cook for 5 minutes, or until onion begins to soften.
4. Add garlic and butternut squash and mix well. Cover skillet and cook for 3 minutes.
5. Make a well in the center of the squash mixture and add ground pork along with sage, rosemary, onion powder, salt, and half of the cinnamon.
6. Break pork up with a spatula as it cooks. Once pork is mostly browned, stir to combine with squash.
7. Cover with a lid and reduce heat to medium-low. Cook for 5-10 minutes, or until the butternut squash is cooked through.
8. Remove lid and add remaining cinnamon. Stir to combine.

Sausage Patties

Adapted from Real Plans
Makes 4 Servings

Ingredients:

1 pound ground pork
1 tablespoon maple syrup, optional
1 teaspoon dried sage
1 teaspoon dried rosemary
1/4 teaspoon cinnamon
1/2 teaspoon fresh ginger
2 teaspoons coarse sea salt
2 tablespoons bacon fat

Directions:

1. Combine all ingredients using clean hands. If possible, allow to sit in the refrigerator overnight or a few hours before cooking.
2. Shape into patties and pan-fry in bacon fat over medium heat until cooked through and slightly browned (about 3-5 minutes per side).

Sheet Pan Greek Chicken and Veggies

From Real Plans
makes 2servings

Ingredients:

4 ounces full fat coconut milk

1 1/2 teaspoons dried oregano

1 1/2 teaspoons lemon juice

1/2 teaspoon sea salt

1 1/2 tablespoons extra virgin olive oil

1/2 pound chicken thigh

parchment paper

1/4 pound Brussels sprouts

1/4 head cauliflower

Directions:

1. In a large bowl, mix together coconut milk, oregano, lemon juice, salt, and 2/3 of the olive oil. Place chicken in the mixture and allow to marinate in the refrigerator for 30-60 minutes.

2. When ready to cook, preheat the oven to 375F. Line a sheet pan with parchment paper. Trim and halve Brussels sprouts. Chop cauliflower.

3. Place Brussels sprouts and cauliflower on one side of the sheet pan. Drizzle with the remaining olive oil and season with salt, to taste. Add chicken to the other side of the sheet pan.

4. Bake for 30-35 minutes, until chicken is cooked through.

5. If desired, turn the oven to broil and broil for 3-5 minutes to crisp up chicken and vegetables.

Shepherd's Pie

From Real Plans
makes 4 servings

Ingredients:

1/2 head cauliflower

6 tablespoons bacon fat, or coconut oil

1 teaspoon coarse sea salt, plus more to taste

1 cup beef broth

1 1/2 tablespoons arrowroot

3 tablespoons filtered water

1 onion

2 carrots

1 pound ground lamb

1 tablespoon fresh parsley

Directions:

1. Preheat oven to 350F.
2. Break the cauliflower into florets.
3. In a large saucepan, cover the cauliflower florets with filtered water and boil until tender. Drain and transfer to a food processor with two-thirds of the fat of choice. Process until cauliflower is smooth. Season with sea salt to taste and set aside.
4. While the cauliflower boils, heat the beef broth in a small saucepan until hot.
5. Mix the arrowroot powder and filtered water together and slowly pour the arrowroot/water mixture into the saucepan of hot broth over low heat. Stir gently until broth thickens into gravy.
6. Dice the onions and carrots.

7. Sauté the onions and carrots with the remaining fat until they begin to soften. Add the ground lamb to brown, breaking apart into small pieces with a wooden spoon.
8. Season with salt to taste.
9. Pour gravy over meat mixture.
10. Transfer the meat mixture into a shallow 2-quart casserole dish. Spoon the cauliflower mash over the meat and spread evenly.
11. Bake for 30 minutes, or until the top is lightly browned. Chop the parsley, sprinkle over the casserole and serve.

Shredded Beef Tacos with Mango Salsa

Adapted from Real Plans
Makes 4 Servings

Ingredients:

1 large mango

1 avocado

1 cucumber

1/2 bunch radish

1/4 small red onion

1 bunch cilantro

1 clove garlic

1 lime

1/2 teaspoon garlic powder

1 teaspoon coarse sea salt, plus more to taste

For the lettuce wraps:

2 cups shredded beef

2 teaspoons coarse sea salt

1 head romaine lettuce, or butter lettuce

2 avocados

2 limes

Directions:

1. For the salsa: Peel and dice the mango, avocado, and cucumber. Dice the radishes. Mince the onion and cilantro. Peel and crush the garlic. Juice the lime.
2. Mix all salsa ingredients in a large bowl.
3. In a food processor, blend about one-third of this mixture until smooth. Reincorporate into the chopped ingredients.
4. If time allows, let the salsa sit (covered) in the fridge for at least an hour or two so the flavors can mingle before serving.

5. For the lettuce wraps: Heat shredded beef on the stovetop until warm. Generously sprinkle with sea salt to taste. If beef wasn't seasoned originally, add onion and garlic powder to taste as well.

6. Remove leaves from the head of lettuce. Rinse and pat dry. Peel, pit, and slice avocados. Slice limes.

7. Fill each leaf with beef, top with salsa and sliced avocado, and garnish with lime.

8. Serve and enjoy.

Shrimp Scampi

Ingredients:

4 zucchini, tops and bottoms cut off, spiralized to make zoodles
1 lb RAW shrimp- peeled and deveined
3 tbsp to ½ cup ghee or coconut oil
1 medium head of garlic- about 10-15 cloves, diced

Directions:

1. In a large pan, melt ghee and add garlic on medium heat.
2. When ghee is melted, add zucchini and shrimp and turn heat to high.
3. Toss zucchini and shrimp often, until shrimp has turned pink.
4. Serve hot!

Note: Ghee is subjective- If you'd like more of a sauce, add a little more. Sometimes you'll have a zucchini that doesn't release as much liquid and you'll need more ghee or coconut oil. Add it slowly as you cook so you can gauge how the recipe is coming together to get a texture you like

Slow Cooker Ham

Adapted from Real Plans
Makes 4 Servings

Ingredients:

2 pounds ham
1/2 cup apple juice
1/2 teaspoon ground ginger
1/4 teaspoon cinnamon
1 cup filtered water

Directions:

1. Place ham in the slow cooker.
2. Combine apple juice, ginger, and cinnamon, then pour over ham. Add water.
3. Slow cook on low for 6 hours.
4. Remove from slow cooker, slice, and serve.

Simple Sauerkraut

Adapted from Real Plans

Ingredients:

4 or 5 heads of red or green cabbage, shredded
1/4 cup sea salt

Directions:

1. Place the shredded cabbage little by little in a fermentation jar (a large, wide-mouth mason jar works great), pounding it vigorously and sprinkling some with the sea salt as you go.
2. Make sure the mixture fills up the jar to no more than 1 inch below the top (because of the expansion), adding more if needed, and that the extracted water covers the vegetables entirely. If it doesn't, create your own brine of 2 tablespoons of sea salt to 4 cups of water and add it to the cabbage.
3. Press the cabbage and keep it under the brine. Cover with a clean towel or cheesecloth to keep out fruit flies. (it is important to not cover with a lid as you need the airflow but don't want bugs.)
4. Place the fermentation jar in a warm spot in your kitchen and allow the sauerkraut to ferment for 7 to 10 days. Check on it from time to time to be sure that the brine covers the vegetables and to remove any mold that may form on the surface. Taste the sauerkraut during the fermentation process, and move it to the refrigerator when you're satisfied with the taste.

Spaghetti Zoodles with Faux-Mato Bolognese

Adapted from Real Plans
Makes 4 Servings

Ingredients:

6 medium zucchinis
1 teaspoon coarse sea salt, plus more for sweating zucchini and to taste
1 small beet
1 onion
5 cloves garlic
3 carrots
1/4 cup fresh basil
3 slices bacon, AIP-friendly
1 cup chicken stock
1 1/2 teaspoons sea salt
1 teaspoon dried oregano
1/2 lemon
2 teaspoons capers
1/4 pound liver, optional
1 pound ground beef

Directions:

1. Preheat your oven to 200F. Use a julienne peeler, a mandolin, a spiralizer, or a very sharp knife to cut the zucchini into ribbons resembling spaghetti. Place the zoodles on a cookie sheet lined with paper towels. Sprinkle with sea salt. "Sweat" the noodles in the oven for 30 minutes until the paper towels have absorbed most of the moisture that the zucchini let. Wrap the paper towels over the noodles and give them a

good squeeze to extract any remaining liquid, and set zoodles aside.

2. Chop beet into one-inch chunks. Boil beet chunks for 10 minutes, or until just tender enough to push a fork all the way through. Strain and set aside.

3. Meanwhile, peel and dice the onion, garlic, carrots, and basil.

4. Saute bacon in a large skillet over low-medium heat until cooked through. Transfer bacon to a plate and reserve bacon grease in the pan. Crumble when cooled.

5. To hot grease, add diced onion and saute for 5 minutes.

6. Add garlic and saute for another 3-4 minutes.

7. Next, add cooked beets, and carrots to the onion and garlic. Saute for 5 minutes then add the crumbled bacon back to the pan.

8. Add chicken stock, salt, and oregano. Simmer 10 minutes, partially covered.

9. Juice the lemon. Pour the entire mixture plus lemon juice and capers into the food processor. Pulse until smooth and the color is red throughout.

10. If you are using liver, remove the veggie mixture from the food processor. Place liver in food processor and pulse until smooth.

11. Add ground beef and liver to the saute pan and cook over medium-high heat until no longer pink (about 5 minutes). Add the faux-mato sauce and chopped basil; simmer 5 minutes more.

12. Add your zoodles to the bolognese sauce, add the fresh basil, and simmer for about 10 minutes.

Stir-Fried Greens with Sausage

Adapted from Real Plans
Makes 4 Servings

Ingredients:

4 tablespoons fish sauce

1 tablespoon coconut aminos

3 cloves garlic

1 1/2 pounds bratwurst, or sausage of choice

1 bunch broccolini, rapine or broccoli

1 bunch kale

4 tablespoons bacon fat, or coconut oil

Directions:

1. In a small bowl, mix the fish sauce and soy sauce. Remove sausage from casing. Mince the garlic.
2. Heat a wok or large skillet over a high flame. Swirl in the oil. Add the sausage and use a wooden spoon to break the meat apart as it browns.
3. Meanwhile, wash the broccolini and shake off excess water. Chop the stalks into 1-inch pieces and set them aside. Chop the leaves into bite-size pieces. Rinse kale and chop into bite-size pieces. Mince the garlic.
4. When the sausage seems about halfway cooked, add the garlic to the pan and stir briefly.
5. If the broccolini stalks are very thick, add them to the pan first, stirring for 1-2 minutes before adding the leaves and kale. Otherwise, add both stalks, leaves, and kale to the pan, followed by the sauce. Stir and toss the vegetables and sausage frequently until the leaves are wilted and the stalks are tender, about 3-5 minutes; serve.

Sunrise Hash

From Real Plans
makes 2 servings

Ingredients:

4 slices bacon
1/2 parsnip
1/2 golden beet, or an extra parsnip
1/2 white sweet potato
1/2 green apple
1/2 head broccoli
1/4 lemon
1/8 teaspoon garlic powder
sea salt, to taste

Directions:

1. Chop the bacon into bite-sized pieces.
2. Heat a large skillet over medium heat. Add the chopped bacon and cook until it has reached its desired crispness. Stir frequently. Once it is cooked, transfer the bacon to a paper towel-lined plate, reserving fat in the pan.
3. Peel and chop the parsnip, beet, and sweet potato. Chop up the apple. Mince the broccoli florets and set them aside. Juice and zest the lemon.
4. Add chopped parsnip, beet, and sweet potato to the hot bacon grease in the pan. Cook 15-20 minutes until vegetables begin to soften.
5. Add the chopped apple. Continue cooking, stirring often, until sweet potatoes are fork-tender. Finally, stir in the broccoli and cooked bacon.
6. Sprinkle in garlic powder. Season with lemon and sea salt.
7. Cook just until the broccoli is a vibrant green. Remove from heat and serve immediately.

Sweet Potato Blueberry Bacon Skillet

Adapted from Real Plans
Makes 2 servings

Ingredients:

2 sweet potatoes
1/2 onion
4 slices bacon
1/2 bunch kale
1 tablespoon extra virgin olive oil, optional
1/2 cup blueberries
1/8 teaspoon ground ginger
sea salt, to taste

Directions:

1. Peel sweet potatoes and cut in half. Cut each half into quarters and then slice in 1/4 inch thick slices. Finely dice the onion and slice bacon slices crosswise. Strip stems from kale and chop into bite-sized pieces.
2. Preheat skillet over medium-high heat and add bacon. Cook until crisp, about 10 minutes.
3. Remove bacon from skillet. Add onions to bacon fat and cook until they begin to soften about 1 minute.
4. Add sweet potatoes to the skillet along with olive oil, if needed. Stir to combine and cover with a lid. Cook, stirring a few times to prevent onions from burning, for 8 minutes, or until potatoes are fork-tender.
5. Remove lid and allow potatoes to cook for 2 more minutes, undisturbed, to crisp a little.
6. Flip potatoes and add kale to the skillet. Stir and allow to wilt down.

7. Add blueberries and ginger; stir to combine and cook for 1 more minute to warm through. Be careful to not overcook, or your breakfast skillet will be blue.
8. Add salt.

Thai Coconut Soup

Adapted from Real Plans
Makes 8 servings

Ingredients:

2 inches ginger
2 stalks lemongrass
12 cups bone broth
2 pounds mushrooms, (oyster shiitake or cremini)
1 lime, zested
8 limes, juiced
1 cup cilantro
4 cups cooked chicken, optional
2 cans full fat coconut milk
8 tablespoons fish sauce, plus more to taste

Directions:

1. Slice ginger into diagonal quarter-inch slices. Cut the lemongrass into 3-inch pieces, and use a pestle or the bottom of a glass ball jar to smash them.
2. Bring stock to a boil in a large saucepan, add ginger and lemongrass, and reduce to a simmer. Continue simmering until stock is reduced to half. Remove ginger and lemongrass.
3. Meanwhile, slice the mushrooms; zest, and juice lime. Chop cilantro, and shred cooked chicken.
4. When the stock is reduced, add lime zest, mushrooms, and coconut milk. Continue simmering for 10-15 minutes, until mushrooms are cooked to desired consistency.
5. Remove from heat. Add shredded chicken. Start seasoning by adding fish sauce and juice of half the limes. Add more fish sauce or lime to taste of either if necessary.
6. Serve steaming, garnished with cilantro.

Thai Crispy Pork Salad

Adapted from Real Plans
Makes 4 Servings

Ingredients:

For the Pork:
2 1/2 pounds pork belly
2 tablespoons fish sauce
1 tablespoon rapadura
For the salad:
1 Granny Smith apple
1 English cucumber
1 head napa cabbage
1 stalk lemongrass
1/2 cup cilantro
For the dressing:
3 cloves garlic
1/2 lime
1 tablespoon maple syrup
1 teaspoon coarse sea salt
2 teaspoons fish sauce, to taste

Directions:

1. Cut pork belly into one-inch wide strips. In a shallow dish, marinate pork belly strips for 4 hours overnight in fish sauce and rapadura.
2. About 2 hours before you're ready to eat, preheat the oven to 350F.
3. Pour off marinade and pat pork belly to dry. Transfer it to a high-sided roasting dish, as quite a bit of fat will render out and spatter.

4. Roast for about 1 hour. At this point, much of the fat should have rendered off, it should be an appetizing golden brown color, and it should be very tender. If it still feels a little firm, give it another half an hour and check again.

5. Meanwhile, prepare the salad and dressing.

6. For the salad: Cut apple into neat matchsticks. Peel cucumber, halve lengthwise, and slice. Slice cabbage and white part of the lemongrass finely. Mince the cilantro. Add all to a large bowl.

7. For the dressing: Peel and chop garlic. Juice the lime. Combine all the dressing ingredients in a small bowl and toss well.

8. Serve hot atop dressed salad.

Tuna Over Kale

Adapted from Real Plans
Makes 4 Servings

Ingredients:

1 onion
1 bunch kale
1 avocado
1 tablespoon olive oil, or coconut oil
10 ounces canned tuna
sea salt, to taste

Directions:

1. Peel and dice onion. Remove stems from kale and roughly chop. Peel, pit, and dice avocado.
2. Heat oil in a pan over medium-high heat. Add onions, and saute until translucent, about 5-7 minutes. Add kale, and cook until starting to wilt. Add tuna, cover, and cook until tuna is warmed through.
3. Top with avocado and salt, to taste. Serve and enjoy!

Turkey and Bacon Rollups

Adapted from Real Plans
Makes 2 Servings

Ingredients:

1 avocado
1 carrot
4 ounces bacon
4 ounces sliced turkey

Directions:

1. Peel, pit, and thinly slice avocado. Shred carrots.
2. Cook bacon in a large heavy-bottomed skillet over medium-high heat until crispy. Remove to a paper towel to drain. Pour bacon fat into a clean mason jar through a fine-mesh strainer to save for cooking later.
3. Lay out the turkey in two-slice layers. In the center of each stack of turkey, place a slice of bacon, a few slivers of avocado, and a sprinkling of shredded carrots.
4. Roll turkey around the filling with seam side down. Slice each roll into 3 pieces and serve.

Veggie Stir Fry with Shrimp

From Real Plans
makes 2 servings

Ingredients:

1 clove garlic
1 tablespoon fresh ginger
1 tablespoon apple cider vinegar
1 tablespoon fish sauce, plus more to taste
1/4 teaspoon honey (optional)
1/2 pound wild shrimp
1/4 head broccoli
1/2 head cauliflower
2 green onions
4 ounces shiitake mushrooms
1 tablespoon coconut oil

Directions:

1. Peel and mince the garlic. Peel and grate the ginger.
2. In a small mixing bowl, add garlic, ginger, apple cider vinegar, fish sauce, and honey. Combine well with a fork or whisk. Set aside.
3. Devein and shell shrimp. Separate broccoli and cauliflower into florets. Mince the green onions finely. Slice the mushrooms.
4. Heat coconut oil over medium-high heat.
5. When the oil is shimmering, add shrimp and mushrooms. Sauté until shrimp start to turn pink but are still slightly translucent.
6. Toss in broccoli and cauliflower. Continue cooking for a minute or two, until the veggies soften.

7. Stir in sauce and cook for an additional minute.
8. Garnish with green onions and serve with extra fish sauce to taste.

Vietnamese Spring Rolls

Adapted from Real Plans
Makes 4 Servings

Ingredients:

12 large shrimp
4 ounces kelp noodles, (Sea Tangle)
1 carrot
1/2 cucumber
1 large avocado
1/2 cup mint leaves
1/2 cup cilantro
1/2 cup fresh basil
1 bunch chives
2 tablespoons coconut oil
1 head butter lettuce
coarse sea salt, to taste
coconut aminos, for dipping

Directions:

1. Bring a large saucepan filled halfway with water to a boil with a generous pinch of sea salt.
2. Devein the shrimp, then drop into the water with heads and tails on.
3. Boil until a few start floating to the top (about 5-7 minutes): Do not overcook or shrimp will be rubbery.
4. Drain the shrimp in a colander, then submerge in an ice bath to stop the cooking process.
5. Remove shells and tails, then slice shrimp in half, lengthwise.
6. For the rolls: To prepare the noodles: Boil kelp noodles for 2 minutes, then drain and cut into two-inch pieces.

7. Peel carrot and cucumber and slice with a mandoline slicer or use a sharp knife to cut as thinly as possible into long matchsticks. Peel and pit avocado; cut into thin slices. Chop the herbs.

8. Place a pinch each of noodles, carrot, cucumber, mint, cilantro, basil, chives, a single row of avocado, and a single row of shrimp onto the center of the wrap. Fold in half like a taco and enjoy.

9. Immediately place a pinch each of noodles, carrot, cucumber, mint, cilantro, basil, chives, a single row of avocado, and a single row of shrimp onto the center of the wrap. Fold bottom then sides of wrap over filling; roll into a cylinder.

10. Serve with coconut aminos for dipping.

Whitefish Packets with Zucchini and Summer Herbs

Adapted from Real Plans
Makes 4 Servings

Ingredients:

4 small zucchinis
1 lemon
2 cloves garlic
4 tablespoons fresh summer herbs, (basil thyme oregano) plus more for garnish
1/4 cup egg-free mayonnaise
1 1/2 pounds red snapper, or other light white fish
2 teaspoons coarse sea salt
parchment paper

Directions:

1. Preheat the oven to 400F.
2. Slice the zucchini into thin 1/8 inch rounds; set aside. Juice the lemon and mince the garlic. Chop fresh herbs.
3. In a small bowl, combine the mayo, lemon juice, garlic, and herbs.
4. Cut fish into individual serving portions. Cut large squares of parchment paper for each serving of fish.
5. Divide the zucchini evenly between the 4 pieces, and place them at the center of each square, topped with a piece of fish. Sprinkle fillet generously with salt.
6. Top each packet with 1/4 of the herb mayo sauce and spread evenly with the back of a spoon.

7. Fold up the parchment paper to make a sealed parcel: With the square sheet in front of you, bring the top and bottom edges together and fold over several times. Then fold each remaining side up to make a neat, tight packet.

8. Bake for 20 minutes. Use a pair of kitchen scissors to cut open the packets, taking care to avoid burns from escaping steam. Garnish with a generous pinch of fresh herbs and serve immediately.

Yolk Ocado

Ingredients:

1 avocado

2 separate egg yolks

Sea salt

Pepper

Directions:

1. Preheat the oven to 425 degrees.
2. Slice the avocado in half, and take out the pit.
3. Place the avocado halve in a small baking dish.
4. Put egg yolk into each avocado half.
5. Bake for 15 to 20 minutes.
6. Remove from oven, and season with sea salt and pepper.

Zucchini Spinach Salad with Chicken

Adapted from Real Plans
Makes 4 Servings

Ingredients:

1/2 lemon
1/4 cup extra virgin olive oil
coarse sea salt, to taste
1 1/4 pounds zucchinis
4 green onions
1/4 cup fresh mint
1 pound cooked chicken
8 ounces baby spinach

Directions:

1. Juice the lemon. In a large bowl, whisk together olive oil, lemon juice, and sea salt to taste.
2. Thinly slice the zucchini. Add the zucchini to the dressing and toss to coat; allow to marinate while preparing the remaining ingredients.
3. Mince the green onions and dice the mint.
4. Shred the chicken and heat it until just until warmed through.
5. Toss the warm chicken with the zucchini mixture. Add spinach, green onions, and mint. Season with sea salt to taste.

Aimee's Butternut Squash Soup

Ingredients:

32 ounces organic butternut squash, cut into 1-inch cubes
4 tablespoons cultured ghee
sea salt
freshly ground black pepper
1 large yellow onion, chopped
3 cloves garlic, minced
5 cups bone broth

Directions:

1. Preheat the oven to 400 degrees. On a foil-lined pan, toss the butternut squash in 2 tbsp of ghee and a pinch of salt and pepper. Roast in the oven for 15 to 20 minutes (depending on the size of the cubes) until the squash is tender. Use a fork to test how tender it is.

2. In a large pot, add the remaining 2 tbsp of ghee and onion, and sauté over medium-high heat for about 10 minutes until the onion has softened. Add the garlic and sauté for an additional minute.

3. Add the roasted butternut squash and the bone broth into the pot. Bring to a simmer. Allow the mixture to simmer for about 5 minutes to let the flavors combine.

4. Turn off the heat and allow the soup to cool for a few minutes. Puree the soup in a blender or food processor. If necessary, do this in several batches; then return the soup to a clean pot. If the soup is too thick for your taste, add a little bit more bone broth. Season with a pinch or two of sea salt.

5. Garnish with fresh cilantro and/or 1/2 an avocado.

Bacon-Beef Liver Pate

From AutoimmuneWellness.com

Ingredients:

6 pieces uncured bacon

1 small onion, minced

4 cloves garlic, minced

1 pound grass-fed beef liver (or chicken liver)

2 tablespoons fresh rosemary, minced

2 tablespoons fresh thyme, minced

½ cup coconut oil, melted

½ teaspoon sea salt

Slices of fresh carrot or cucumber (omit when in Phase 2)

Directions:

1. Cook the bacon slices in a cast-iron pot until crispy. Set aside to cool, reserving the grease in the pan to cook the liver.
2. Add the onion and cook for 2 minutes on medium-high. Add the garlic and cook for a minute. Add the liver, sprinkling with the herbs. Cook for 3-5 minutes per side, until no longer pink in the center.
3. Turn off heat, and place contents into a blender or food processor with the coconut oil and sea salt. Process until it forms a thick paste, adding more coconut oil if too thick.
4. Cut the cooled bacon strips into little bits and mix with the pâté in a small bowl. Garnish with some fresh herbs and serve on carrot or cucumber slices.

Coconut Yogurt

Yield: 2 to 3 servings

Ingredients

1 BPA-free can of full-fat coconut milk, 13.5 ounces

1 tablespoon fermented coconut-water probiotic kefir,
or 1 capsule of any probiotic to use as your starter

½ teaspoon of organic ground cinnamon

Directions

1. For thicker yogurt, refrigerate the can of coconut milk (don't shake it up) for at least 3 hours so that the cream rises to the top. Then use just the cream, not the water, at the bottom of the can. If you prefer a thinner yogurt, use the entire can of coconut milk—water and all. The amount of yogurt you get from this recipe is equal to the amount of coconut milk you use. So if you use an entire 13.5-ounce can, you'll get the whole 13.5 ounces, or about 1 ¾ cups.

2. Place the coconut milk, or just the cream if you choose, into a sterilized glass jar with either the tablespoon of kefir or the contents of the probiotic capsule. If you're working with the probiotic capsule, open it up and dump in the powder. Then mix with a plastic or metal spoon.

3. Put the sealed jar of yogurt in the oven with the light on. DO NOT TURN THE OVEN ON. Just close the oven door and turn on the oven light. A closed oven with the light on will generate a stable temperature of about 105° to 110°F, perfect conditions for the coconut milk to incubate. The longer it sits, the more yogurt-y it becomes, so I leave mine in for 24 hours. Normally, you'd let dairy milk sit for 7 hours after heating it up on the stove to get it to that 110°F, but I'm using a

shortened preparation process. It's not necessary to heat up either dairy milk or coconut milk before letting it incubate. The yogurt may still be watery; if so, put it in the refrigerator for a few hours to help it solidify. Before eating, sprinkle it with cinnamon.

Ginger Turmeric Bone Broth

Yields 10-12 servings

Ingredients

¼ teaspoon mustard seeds

2 teaspoon cumin seeds (or 1 teaspoon ground)

2 teaspoon coriander seeds (or 1 teaspoon ground)

2 tablespoons cultured ghee

1 onion, diced

1 piece lemongrass (remove outer hull, bruise the remaining layers with a knife, and chop finely)

1 ½ tablespoons ginger, finely chopped (or 2 teaspoons ground)

1 ½ tablespoons freshly grated turmeric (or 2 teaspoons ground)

4 garlic cloves, minced

4 cups filtered water

4 cups bone broth

1 teaspoon sea salt

2 teaspoons apple cider vinegar

A few sprigs of cilantro, for garnish

Scallions, chopped, for garnish

A few sprigs of mint, for garnish

1 avocado, diced, for garnish

Directions

1. Crush the mustard seeds, cumin seeds, and coriander seeds with a mortar and pestle (or spice grinder) as finely as possible. If using ground spices, then skip this step.
2. In a large, heavy-bottomed pot or Dutch oven, heat the ghee over medium-high heat.

3. Add the onion and sauté for 5 minutes. Add the lemongrass, ginger, and fresh turmeric and lower the heat to medium. Sauté for 5 minutes until it all starts to brown, stirring often.
4. Add the garlic and sauté for 2 more minutes.
5. Add the ground spices and sauté for 1 more minute.
6. Add the water, bone broth, and salt and bring to a simmer.
7. Add the apple cider vinegar.
8. Adjust your seasonings to taste. Garnish with cilantro, scallions, mint, and avocado.
9. Reserve in the refrigerator. Break the soup up into batches (I use 12-ounce mason jars) and freeze most of the broth immediately, leaving in the fridge only what you will consume over the next 2 to 3 days.

References

1 PLOS Genetics. 2012; D. C. Woods, E. E. Telfer, J. L. Tilly. https://doi.org/10.1371/journal.pgen.1002848

2 Ageing Res Rev 2020 Nov;63:101168. doi: 10.1016/j.arr.2020.101168. Epub 2020 Sep 4

3 Crit Rev Biochem Mol Biol. 2019 Feb; 54(1): 61–83. doi: 10.1080/10409238.2019.1570075

4 Sci Rep. 2017; 7: 1434. doi: 10.1038/s41598-017-01609-3

5 Front Endocrinol (Lausanne). 2019; 10: 346. https://www.ncbi.nlm.nih.gov/pmc/articles/PMC6568019/

6 Adv Exp Med Biol. 2020;1247:109-123. doi: 10.1007/5584_2019_456. https://pubmed.ncbi.nlm.nih.gov/31802446/

7 https://doi.org/10.18632/aging.202913

8 https://doi.org/10.1111/j.1439-0531.2012.02086.x

9 J Clin Invest. 2008 Apr 1; 118(4): 1210; doi: 10.1172/JCI35350

10 JAMA Intern Med. 2018;178(1):17-26. doi:10.1001/jamainternmed.2017.5038

11 Aging Cell 2012 Dec;11(6):1046-54. doi: 10.1111/acel.12006. Epub 2012 Oct 19.

12 https://www.preventmiscarriage.com/no-benefit-found-with-intralipid-therapy-ground-.html

13 Raupp, Aimee: Yes, You Can Get Pregnant (2014); Demos Health

14 Shanahan, C, M.D., Deep Nutrition: Why Your Genes Need Traditional Foods. 2008. Flatiron Books.

15 Fertility and Sterility: 2012, 98 (3), S
  47;I:https://doi.org/10.1016/j.fertnstert.2012.07.167

16 https://www.thepaleomom.com/reintroducing-foods-after-
  following-the-autoimmune-protocol/

Printed in Great Britain
by Amazon

21671811R00203